# IRRITABLE BOWEL SYNDROME

THIRD EDITION

# IRRITABLE BOWEL SYNDROME

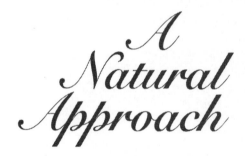

*A Natural Approach*

**ROSEMARY NICOL**

FOREWORD BY WILLIAM JOHN SNAPE, JR., M.D.

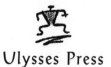

Ulysses Press

Published by: Ulysses Press
P.O. Box 3440
Berkeley, CA 94703
www.ulyssespress.com

ISBN10: 1-56975-602-3
ISBN13: 978-1-56975-602-7
Library of Congress Catalog Contr

First published as *Coping Successfully with Your Irritable Bowel,*
*The Irritable Bowel Stress Book,* and *The Irritable Bowel Diet Book*
by Sheldon Press

Printed in Canada by Transcontinental Printing

20  19  18  17  16  15  14  13  12  11  10  9

Update Author: William John Snape, Jr., M.D.
Editor: Mark Woodworth
Cover Design: Double R Design
Interior Illustrations: Claudine Gossett
Editorial and production staff: Claire Chun, Matt Orendorff,
   Elyce Petker, Ruth Marcus
Indexer: Sayre Van Young

Distributed by Publishers Group West

The author and publisher welcome
your comments and suggestions for future editions.
We would also appreciate hearing how this book has helped you.
Please write us at Ulysses Press, P.O. Box 3440, Berkeley, CA
94703. You can also e-mail us at readermail@ulyssespress.com.

# *Contents*

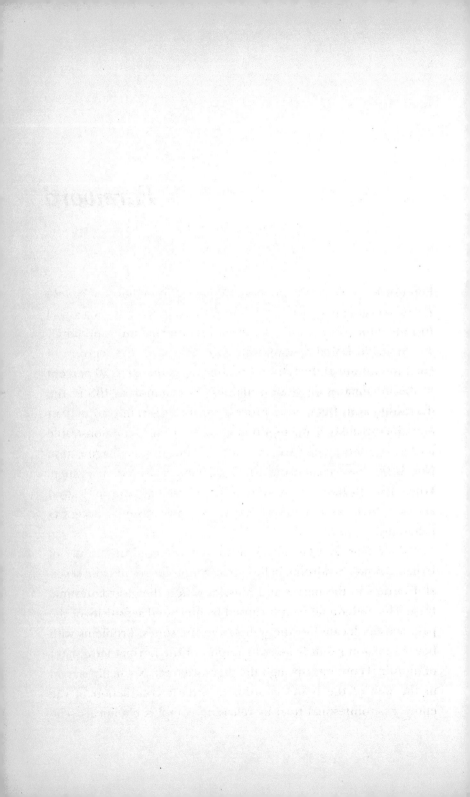

# *Foreword*

It is a pleasure to see the publication of the third edition of *Irritable Bowel Syndrome*—a book that will be a worthwhile support to medical treatment for patients suffering from this often painful condition.

Irritable Bowel Syndrome is a general term for a group of common intestinal tract disorders affecting some 20 to 30 percent of the inhabitants of western nations. As common as IBS is, the diagnostic and therapeutic process can be frustrating to patient and doctor alike. Patients do not suffer from a demonstrable anatomic abnormality that can be seen during an imaging test. Nor do they have an abnormality that can be measured on a gauge. What they do have are symptoms of abdominal pain and alterations of their bowel habit, which we as physicians must accept at face value.

Physicians actively involved in determining the cause of Irritable Bowel Syndrome believe that symptoms result from several disorders in the nerves and muscles within the gastrointestinal tract. The abdominal pain is caused by increased sensitivity of the pain sensors located in the wall of the intestines. Problems with bowel function result from a disruption of the normal movement of intestinal contents through the digestive tract. Normally, nerves in the wall of the bowel coordinate orderly contraction of the entire gastrointestinal tract by releasing complex chemicals. The brain's response to emotional stress initiates additional nerve signals that alter these chemical regulators.

Successful medical therapy for Irritable Bowel Syndrome involves 1) altering the diet or reducing stress levels, thereby modifying the input to the nerves in the wall of the colon from the brain or other parts of the bowel, 2) decreasing the sensitivity of the nerves in the wall of the bowel, or 3) directly altering the contractile response of the muscle lining of the intestine. After identifying the specific disturbance that leads to the patient's symptoms, the physician can initiate the best therapy. This book outlines appropriate lifestyle changes, which may also reduce IBS symptoms and benefit the patient.

The quandary faced by many patients is demonstrated in the book by one of my patients. Mrs. G, a middle-aged woman, has suffered from cramping pain in her lower abdomen for many years, along with an associated change in bowel habit. Eating and emotional stress make this pain worse. She has been seen by many physicians, who completed uncomfortable and expensive work-ups, which revealed no physical abnormality. She cancels many work, social and household activities because of her symptoms. Her excuse for each of the cancellations is abdominal discomfort. Her emotional state rises or sinks depending on whether her family and friends believe her symptoms to be real or fabricated. Her anger, frustration and anxiety levels increase during discussions with her harried physician, who lacks the time or inclination to explain the physical or psychological causes of her symptoms. She is distraught when the physician implies that her symptoms are purely psychological and without a physical basis. This book provides patients such as Mrs. G. both comfort in knowing that they are not alone in their problem and the information needed to understand the anatomy and the function of their gastrointestinal tract and how it reacts to psychological stress. The words used to describe the body's functions are clearly defined so the patient has the best chance to understand his or her physician.

*Irritable Bowel Syndrome* offers patients diagnosed with IBS a clear explanation of the mechanisms causing their symptoms. I hope that this knowledge will also provide sufferers reassurance that their illness is not life threatening.

The book also provides the patient with a broad range of therapeutic options. These range from the conventional to less accepted alternative methods. However, *Irritable Bowel Syndrome* has two underlying themes that are particularly helpful to the patient seeking adequate relief of IBS symptoms. First, there must be a realistic acceptance of the goals of therapy; and, second, there is much that patients can do to help themselves. I believe the patient and the physician have been successful if the patient's symptoms have been more than 80 percent relieved, and the patient is able to fulfill all the functions of daily life. And the physician should feel pleased if the patient contributes to his or her treatment by making positive lifestyle changes: limiting emotional stress, changing eating habits, and avoiding the toxic effects of cigarettes, alcohol, and caffeine. These patients will be empowered to enter into a partnership with their physician to improve their symptoms. This teamwork approach to good health will be a win-win situation for both doctor and patient.

—William John Snape, Jr., M.D.

# *Acknowledgments*

I would like to acknowledge my gratitude for the invaluable help given to me in the writing of this book. In particular my deepest thanks must go to:

Mr. Andrew Gough, Consultant Surgeon, Weston General Hospital, Weston-super-Mare, who gave me so much of his time with help and information; and Dr. Enid Smith, General Practitioner, who also answered questions and gave help when I needed it.

In addition, I would like to thank the following people who gave help so willingly: Dr. Ken Heaton, Reader in Medicine, University of Bristol Department of Medicine; Dr. Rosalind Hinton, Member of the British Society of Medical and Dental Hypnosis; Mr. Ian MacGregor, Member of the National Institute of Medical Herbalists; Mrs. Therese Parsons, Member of the Traditional Acupuncture Society; Mr. Steve Sandler, Registered Osteopath, Director of Osteopathic Practice at the British School of Osteopathy; Dr. Jeremy Swayne, Homeopathic Physician, Regional Tutor of the Faculty of Homeopathic Medicine; and Dr. John Hunter, Consultant Physician, Gastro-enterology Research Unit, Addenbrooke's Hospital, Cambridge, and his publishers, Macdonald, for permission to use the exclusion diet, and to reproduce the table.

Finally, I would like to express my gratitude to my husband, David, for all his help and support; to our children for their tolerance and encouragement, especially our eldest daughter, Katie, who provided me with so much information on food and diet; and to the many people who shared with me their personal experience of living with Irritable Bowel Syndrome.

# *Introduction*

You are probably reading this book because you have a condition called Irritable Bowel Syndrome. You may know one or two other people who have it too. But I expect it isn't something you like to talk about very much. It doesn't often come up in polite conversation; people don't usually compare their irritable bowels over drinks or dinner. The very description of the condition, containing as it does the word *bowel*, tends to keep it rather private.

Yet about one-third of the population has had the symptoms of Irritable Bowel Syndrome (IBS) at some time or another, and about 20 to 30 percent of the general population has them regularly. That's a lot of people, and this percentage is common throughout most of the Western world. Nearly half of all the patients that most gastroenterologists see in hospital outpatient departments present symptoms of IBS. So there's a lot of it around—you are not alone.

It would seem reasonable, therefore, to expect IBS to be better known. There are two possible reasons why it isn't. First, we have a natural reluctance to discuss anything to do with the body's nether regions. Most of us were brought up to regard bodily functions as somewhat dirty and faintly disgusting. We were taught to keep them out of sight and out of mind. Anything to do with bowels, bowel movements, and related matters is definitely not a polite subject in our clean Western culture. Because bowel matters are so little talked about, people often silently suffer discomfort, distress, and embarrassment. This is a pity, because we all (from the highest in the land to the lowest) have bowel movements, and the way our bowels function is important to our health.

The second reason why Irritable Bowel Syndrome is not generally mentioned is, I suspect, because of its name. To be honest, the words *irritable* and *bowel* do not exactly conjure up the sort of image most people would like to have of themselves. If it were called something like "Intestinal Motility Disorder," "Functional Colon Disease," or "Thingamajig's Syndrome," it might have a better public image. Some medical books do call IBS by different names—"Irritable Colon," "Spastic Colon," "Mucus Colitis," "Spastic Colitis," even "Tense Tummy"—but none of these has slipped into common usage. So until someone decides on a change of name, we are stuck with Irritable Bowel Syndrome, and I hope that by the time you finish reading this book you will have overcome any embarrassment you might have concerning digestive functions, their names, and their descriptions.

—Rosemary Nicol

# 1

# *What Is Irritable Bowel Syndrome?*

## Who Gets Irritable Bowel Syndrome?

Anybody can get IBS—you, me, Peter at work, Jane next door. Just because friends and co-workers don't talk about it doesn't mean they don't have it. In fact, 15 to 20 percent of the general population have symptoms consistent with IBS—that's more than 35 million people.

When people asked me what I was writing a book about, and I replied, "Irritable Bowel Syndrome," I was amazed at how many people said, "I get that." Often they were people I'd known for a long time; I knew about their families, their jobs, their holiday plans, their illnesses, even their political and religious beliefs, but I didn't know about their irritable bowels. Most people keep such information very much to themselves.

So who is most likely to get it? Usually, people who suffer from IBS have recently undergone a period of stress—the breakup of a relationship, a layoff from work, money worries, or other related difficulties. In fact, 51 percent of IBS patients have noted a stressful event preceding their bout with IBS. Also, people who have IBS tend to live such busy lives that they don't make time to eat meals in a calm, relaxed way.

IBS sufferers often experience their first symptoms in late adolescence or early adulthood. About twice as many women as men suffer from IBS, and most people with the condition are between 20 and 40 years old.

People who get IBS often fall into two extremes: At one extreme are healthy and robust individuals who never see a doctor about it and don't feel it upsets their lives in any way. They get it from time to time, but it hardly bothers them. At the other extreme are those for whom IBS is devastating. They dare not move far from a toilet; they feel isolated, panicky, totally lacking in self-confidence. Their social life is ruined, their diet is horribly restricted, and they worry that their poor health may cause them to lose their job. Their tummy becomes the center of the universe, and they live in fear of the tricks their bodies may have in store for them. In between are the great majority, who manage quite well most of the time but still have to watch what they eat and find that their guts get the better of them if they get tense or agitated.

If you don't like the effect IBS has on your life, take *comfort*. There's a lot you can do about it. If the pills and medicines you get from the doctor don't work as well as you'd like, there are plenty of other things you can try. Be prepared to make some changes, to take a new look at yourself, to accept that your health may be in your own hands, and to say, "From today on I am going to make me better."

---

## IBS FACTS

- 8–17 percent of the population has IBS
- Women with IBS outnumber men 2 to 1
- Only the common cold accounts for more sick days
- Stress triggers about half of all episodes of IBS

source: "Bowels in an Uproar," *Johns Hopkins Magazine*

## What Exactly Is Irritable Bowel Syndrome?

IBS is a disorder of

1. The way in which the food you eat moves through the 30-plus feet of tubing that makes up the large and small intestines. (See the diagram on page 23, and also pages 18–21 for definitions of medical terms you may come across in this book.)

2. The way these intestines react to various things, particularly diet and stress.

How and why this happens, and what you can do about it, is the subject of this book.

## What Are the Symptoms of IBS?

For years, patients suffered in silence or went to their doctors with an odd assortment of symptoms that nowadays are recognized as typical of Irritable Bowel Syndrome. These are

—Abdominal pain (pain in the tummy), usually low down on the left, or possibly center or right

—Diarrhea, with or without stomach pain

—Constipation, usually with stomach pain, and small, lumpy stools like "rabbit droppings"

—Alternating diarrhea and constipation, often in an unpredictable and erratic pattern

—An abdomen that looks or feels bloated and distended

—Feeling "full of gas"

—Passing mucus with the stools or by itself

In addition, IBS generally becomes worse during periods of stress and may disappear completely at other times.

This particular collection of symptoms is found only in Irritable Bowel Syndrome. Most people with IBS have several of them, particularly abdominal pain, along with a tummy that feels distended and a bowel-movement pattern that varies. People with other conditions very seldom have more than two or three of the symptoms.

In addition, if you have IBS, it is quite likely that you will have some of the lesser symptoms from the following list:

DIGESTIVE

Heartburn

Nausea

Feeling full early in a meal

Unpleasant taste in the mouth

Loss of appetite

Regurgitating acid

Belching

Difficulty swallowing

Rumblings and gurglings (borborygmus)

Occasional vomiting

BOWEL AND BLADDER

Passing urine often

Urgently needing to go to the toilet

After a bowel movement feeling there is more stool to come

STATES OF MIND

Tiredness or lethargy

Anxiety

Irritation

Loss of concentration

Mild depression and weeping

Lack of "sparkle"

## PHYSICAL

Back pain

Sleeping difficulties

Feeling hot behind the eyes (like flu)

Headache, possibly with sweating, flushes, and faintness

Reduced sex drive

## EXTRA PROBLEMS FOR WOMEN

Painful sexual intercourse

Painful menstrual periods

It's hardly surprising that, with many of these widely varying complaints, doctors used to think IBS patients were hypochondriacs! But they aren't, and these complaints are now recognized as being extremely common with IBS. Many of them are linked with constipation, so by getting rid of your constipation you might also get rid of some of the undesirable extras.

In addition, people with IBS are often worried by

—*Seeing recognizable food in their stools*—this is because some food has not been properly digested

—*Rumblings and gurglings*—which just mean that the digestive process is happening

—*Passing mucus*—this is not a symptom of disease, just of the bowel being overly sensitive

—*Fear of cancer*—as you will read more than once in this book, there is no known connection between IBS and bowel cancer.

## What Causes Irritable Bowel Syndrome?

Most people can trace their Irritable Bowel Syndrome back to

—An attack of viral or bacterial gastroenteritis, which may make the intestines overreactive and sensitive

—A long or strong course of antibiotics, which may alter the delicate balance of natural beneficial bacteria in the body

—An abdominal or pelvic operation

—A stressful time such as divorce, threat of job layoff, unemployment, exams, and so on

A previous bowel infection may cause symptoms by inducing a chronic bacterial growth in the small intestine or may initiate a low-grade inflammatory process in the bowel wall. Pelvic operations are especially prone to cause symptoms of Irritable Bowel Syndrome. A hysterectomy removes one of the stabilizing forces for the pelvic floor.

Some foods aggravate IBS symptoms, but food is probably not the original cause of the syndrome.

Using irritating laxatives too often is another major cause of IBS. Some people hold the mistaken belief that a daily emptying of the bowels is essential to good health. Also, many people with IBS frequently ignore the normal urge to have a bowel movement, which irritates their bowels further.

From this, you can see that IBS is caused by circumstantial conditions. If you can eat food that does not upset you, if you can avoid laxatives, and if you can learn to reduce stress or at least cope more effectively with the stress you have, then you are less likely to suffer from an irritable bowel.

Before you say to yourself, "Well, it's too late now, I've got it," *don't despair*. As various aspects of your life probably triggered IBS in the first place, it is likely that, by making some changes in the way you live, you can live with it, come to terms with it, and perhaps eliminate it altogether.

I hope that after reading this chapter you have been reassured that you are quite normal, like all those other individuals who have IBS. You may have an odd assortment of complaints, but they are all part of this particular syndrome. So read on and discover how you can greatly relieve it and possibly be rid of it forever.

## How Can I Tell If I Have It?

When you have eliminated the impossible, whatever remains . . . must be the truth.

—Sherlock Holmes, *The Sign of the Four*

Until quite recently, diagnosis of IBS was rather like Sherlock Holmes' famous statement. When presented with patients with chronic, recurring stomach pain plus assorted other symptoms, doctors would carry out various tests and investigations for numerous diseases. When all the tests proved negative, the doctors would pronounce their verdict: "There's nothing wrong with you," or just possibly, "You haven't got anything particular, therefore you have Irritable Bowel Syndrome."

This approach was not ideal. For a start, all those consultations and tests were expensive and time consuming. Then, the doctors' continuing failure to diagnose anything "real" tended to weaken patients' confidence in them. The time taken to undergo tests and then wait for negative results was dispiriting for the patient. When the final verdict was pronounced, neither doctor nor patient necessarily had confidence in it. "The doctor couldn't think what else it might be, so he just said I had Irritable Bowel Syndrome and I must learn to live with it."

The problem was that, unlike most diseases, IBS had no real set of clues to aid diagnosis. If you have chicken pox or mumps or a peptic ulcer, or almost any other gastrointestinal disease, it can be diagnosed from well-established guidelines. Your doctor can ask questions, examine you, do tests, and come to a firm and confident conclusion.

IBS is not like that. It is not an organic disease, yet it mimics many other organic diseases. In fact, one of the guidelines to a correct diagnosis of IBS is that there is no evidence of any organic disease. You may have certain symptoms that might well be disease A, B, or C, yet you clearly do not have these diseases; that in itself is a indicator of IBS for the doctor. But IBS is not just a "diagnosis of exclusion"; that is, when other diseases are excluded, you must have the only thing left—Irritable Bowel Syndrome. There are now several clearly defined symptoms that, if you have them, mean you have IBS.

Before we look at these symptoms, it's worth looking at the problems of diagnosis from your doctor's viewpoint. Her patient has the sort of symptoms that could, on first appearance, be any one of a number of diseases. The persistent pain, the distended abdomen, the alternating constipation and diarrhea, and the assorted other symptoms (headache, tiredness, nausea, back pain) could all be caused by something that she mustn't overlook. In addition, her patient may be fearful that she has cancer or some serious bowel disorder. It is obviously most important that the doctor not miss anything.

Because of this, many doctors used to be tempted to try a "shotgun" approach—that is, arrange tests and investigations for every conceivable disorder and hope that one of them shows something. This can reflect a doctor's uncertainty and can undermine the relationship between doctor and patient, since the more tests the doctor carries out the more anxious the patient is likely to become.

Fortunately, this is no longer necessary. Thanks to a lot of research that has been done on the irritable bowel, there are now clear guidelines for diagnosis. If you, the sufferer, are aware of these guidelines, you are more likely to believe your doctor when he tells you that you have Irritable Bowel Syndrome. Having believed him, you will be in a good position to work toward coping with it.

IBS is not a physical disease; it is a disorder in the functioning of part of the digestive system. It is unlikely to get much worse, but for some people it may never get completely better. Once you can accept that and learn how to manage it, you will find it much easier to live with. Rest assured that there is no known link between IBS and cancer of the digestive system, nor is IBS life threatening. It may cause you pain, inconvenience, and even distress, but it will not kill you.

If the following circumstances describe your condition, you can be confident that you have Irritable Bowel Syndrome and not some other disease. People with other disorders seldom have more than two or three symptoms at most. (See pages 18–21 for any medical terms you don't understand.)

1. The more of the following symptoms you have, the more likely it is that you have IBS:

   • Abdominal pain that is relieved by having a bowel movement

   • Loose stools when the pain starts

   • More frequent stools when the pain starts

   • Small, dry stools like "rabbit droppings"

   • Alternating diarrhea and constipation

   • Bloating and distension of the abdomen, often with gas

   • The feeling after a bowel movement that there is more stool to come

   • Passing mucus with stools

2. You have had a sigmoidoscopy, barium enema, blood tests, and a rectal examination and they all prove normal. If you are under 40, and other tests are normal, your doctor may decide the sigmoidoscopy and barium enema are not necessary. (You will read more about these tests in Chapter 2.)

3. You have no serious loss of weight, you do not pass blood in your stools, and you have had the symptoms for quite a long time (two years or more).

If your doctor has taken a detailed medical history from you, and these three conditions apply, and he now tells you that you have Irritable Bowel Syndrome, then it is highly likely that you can have confidence in his diagnosis.

So IBS *is*

—A problem of how your insides work

—A disorder in the way food moves through the intestines

—A condition aggravated by stress or the wrong diet

—A condition that comes and goes

—A condition that is tiresome but surprisingly common

And IBS *is not*

—Cancer or any cancer-related disease

—Inflammatory bowel disease, ulcerative colitis, Crohn's disease, or any other serious bowel disease

—An organic disease

—A life-threatening disease

—A disease suffered only by neurotics and hypochondriacs

If you are under 40 (say, mid to late 30s), it is highly unlikely that you have cancer of the colon or rectum. If you are over 40, the doctor will probably check for these. If the tests come back negative, then rest assured. As I have mentioned before, there is no documented mortality or serious disease connected with IBS. Since so many people with IBS fear they may have cancer, it is important for you to know whether you do or not. Bowel cancer kills more people in the Western world than any other cancer except lung cancer, yet it has a good cure rate if it is detected early.

As you can see, a positive diagnosis of IBS does involve a doctor; you cannot be totally confident without her or his help. For this reason, if you think you may have IBS (or any other medical condition), it is important to get it correctly diagnosed by a doctor. Don't rush straight into self-treatment—you may overlook something serious.

If you are worried, see a doctor as soon as possible. If you do have cancer or some other very serious disease, you will greatly increase your chances of recovery; if your doctor says that you have Irritable Bowel Syndrome, trust the diagnosis and read the rest of this book.

## "It's All In Your Mind, Mrs. Jones"

But it isn't, is it? It's right there, in your insides, only other people don't really believe you. Instead, they tell you that if only you'd pull yourself together, stop worrying about it, and join an evening class, all your symptoms would disappear. And everybody (your doctor, your family and friends) could have a quiet life.

While researching this book, I read several dozen articles in highly reputable medical journals, and the same words kept cropping up: *neurotic, aggressive, anxious, depressed, obsessive.* There is little doubt that many doctors still regard these words as the classic descriptors of someone with an irritable bowel, so they tell their patients that the symptoms are due to their nerves and are largely imaginary (or at least greatly exaggerated), and then prescribe tranquilizers.

Now you know this is unjust, but why do some doctors not see that? To be fair to them, there is little doubt that many people with Irritable Bowel Syndrome who visit their doctor tend to have more general complaints than the population at large. They are more likely to see the doctor for a cold or flu than to treat such conditions themselves. They are more likely to have days off work, headaches, and sleep difficulties. They often have more problems at work, anxiety over their children or their parents, and concern about their marriage. They tend to worry more about small problems than most people do. In general, these particular people are more likely to visit doctors than to take responsibility for their own health. They also have a greater fear of cancer and other serious diseases, and the anxiety that this generates may aggravate their IBS symptoms.

Yet doctors are seeing a self-selected group: those who have decided to visit the doctor. This group is not typical. The vast majority of people with IBS do not see a doctor at all; they don't regard their condition as serious or abnormal in any way, and they are in other respects robust, healthy people. They seek no advice and do not bring their condition to the doctor's attention.

So people who do see the doctor about their irritable bowel are a small group, not typical of the majority. And those who progress beyond the doctors, who go on to visit hospital specialists and volunteer for IBS research projects and drug trials (which are then written up in professional journals) are a smaller group still. Many researchers mistakenly assume that the people they see in hospital surveys are typical. They then assume that what they have discovered in a small, self-selected, and atypical group applies to everyone with IBS, even to those who seek no medical help.

Although people with IBS make up about half the patients seen by most gastroenterologists, it is quite unfair to label everyone with this condition as neurotic or overanxious. Twenty to thirty percent of apparently healthy people in the United States have IBS, yet the great majority seek help only from their general practitioners or not at all.

So let us now look at why some doctors put these rather unattractive labels on so many people. A fictitious patient (let's call her Mrs. Jones) visits the doctor again. She's already been many times before, usually about a pain in her abdomen, though she also has headaches, gas, and sleeping problems, and she does seem rather anxious about things in general.

The doctor's heart sinks when he sees her. "What is it this time?" he thinks to himself. He has prescribed a variety of medicines for her (none of which have had much success); he's examined her and found nothing wrong; he's referred her to the specialist, who also found nothing wrong; and the specialist arranged for her to have some tests, which all proved normal. If there is nothing wrong with her, surely she must be imagining things. He has a waiting room full of people with conditions that respond positively to his treatments, and, quite honestly, he is beginning to lose patience with Mrs. Jones. So he tells her she has Irritable Bowel Syndrome (which should satisfy her need for a diagnosis), says she must stop worrying about things, and prescribes some tranquilizers to calm her down, plus some antispasmodics and a bulk laxative.

Looking at it objectively, the doctor's viewpoint does not seem unreasonable, does it? From Mrs. Jones's viewpoint, however, things look rather different. She's had a pain in her tummy for quite a long time, together with bowel habits that are quite variable—sometimes constipation, sometimes diarrhea. She feels full of gas, too, but the problem that most concerns her is her tummy ache. Nothing seems to make it better. She's tried indigestion tablets, laxatives, and a whole range of painkillers, and still it never goes away for long. In Mrs. Jones's mind, a pain that never really gets better and that doesn't respond to painkillers is worrisome. Could it be something serious, like cancer? She sees her doctor, who prescribes medicines that don't work. She gets more worried. The doctor sends her to the hospital for various tests, all of which conclude that there is nothing wrong with her. But there *must* be something wrong. Why does she keep getting this pain and such topsy-turvy bowel habits? Is the doctor keeping some dreadful truth from her? Should she perhaps find a different doctor?

Poor Mrs. Jones. To have symptoms that distress her and reduce the quality of her life is bad enough. Worse still to find that no one seems to know what causes them. And the last straw is to realize that her doctor thinks she's making it all up.

I know that I am being unfair to many doctors who do know about IBS. Although they realize that IBS can be stress related, they also know it has clearly recognized physical causes. They reassure their patients, take time to explain the condition to them, and prescribe treatments, such as a high-fiber diet and antispasmodic medicines, that will almost certainly work.

However, most doctors often treat only the symptoms of IBS without taking time to discover the underlying causes of stress and (in some cases) diet. If doctors could help patients to identify and manage stress and to eat proper food, they would probably see their IBS patients less frequently. But how many busy doctors can find time to teach relaxation and work out individual diet sheets? And should that really be part of a doctor's job?

Recognizing that IBS is not "all in the mind" is half the battle. There are indeed physical causes, and, to be fair to your unsympathetic doctor, many of these physical causes are aggravated by states of mind.

You will almost certainly have noticed that, when you are slightly nervous or anxious about anything, you get "butterflies" in your tummy. You may also need to go to the toilet more often, and you possibly don't feel much like eating. These are quite normal reactions, and they occur because there are direct nerve pathways between the brain and the gut. Quite simply, how your mind feels affects how your stomach behaves, and, conversely, if your stomach is churned up your mind will be churned up, too. There is nothing unusual about this. When you are under stress of any kind, your stomach will produce more hydrochloric acid, which causes your bowel to contract more vigorously than normal.

If you have IBS you may also have other physical conditions that trigger your delicate gut:

—You probably have some abnormality in the way the muscle of your large intestine propels its contents. This abnormality is either inherited or caused by previous gastrointestinal infections. Because of this, your muscles are likely to contract more vigorously than normal, causing spasm and pain.

—The muscles of your intestines may be extrasensitive.

—You may produce more mucus than usual.

—Gastroenteritis or a long course of antibiotics can cause changes to take place in the useful bacteria that live in the gut and that help in the normal process of digestion. Candida albicans, which may be a factor in IBS, favors these conditions.

—Different foods cause the intestines to produce different chemicals, and your gut may overreact to some of these chemicals with more contractions and increased sensitivity.

—Pain is not measurable scientifically—we all feel it at different levels. What is mild discomfort to one person may be severe pain to another. Perhaps some people with IBS have particularly low thresholds of pain.

—Almost certainly, the nature of your bowel means that you feel more pain than usual when the lower bowel (the rectum) is full, as in constipation. This fullness in the bowel may produce pain the most unlikely places: the back, shoulders, thigh, and the area around the anus.

—If you have diarrhea as a main symptom, you may have an "incompetent sigmoid colon," which means that the last part of the colon does not work as well as it should. This allows sloppy contents to descend into the rectum before all the water has been absorbed.

These physical causes are real and recognizable and are not just "all in your mind." They can be treated. Firstly, if your bowel muscles contract more vigorously than usual, it is important to make sure the contents of the bowel are soft and bulky, not hard and small. And if your lower bowel feels pain when it is full then try to empty you bowels more often. The answer to both of these conditions is to eat a diet with plenty of fiber and to make sure you do not become constipated.

If you get a lot of diarrhea, it may well be from stress, but it could also be from a clear physical cause: your body may not produce enough of the enzyme lactase to digest the milk products you eat. If you are referred to a gastroenterologist, this is one of the tests he or she may arrange for you. If it turns out that you do have some intolerance to milk products, you would be well advised to consume less of them.

Again, the solution to so many of your digestive problems is in your own hands and not necessarily in more medicines. Rather than ask yourself, What shall I take for this? ask, What can I do about this?

Finally, let us suppose that your IBS does cause you to be difficult to live with at times. Is this really surprising? The very nature of IBS can reduce your self-confidence. Having continuing pain will obviously affect the quality of your life. Always having to watch what you eat can play havoc with your social life, and the constant need to be near a toilet does nothing for your self-esteem. Having chronic symptoms that doctors cannot diagnose is worrying. The need to discuss bowels and bowel movements is distasteful to many people, as is the thought of being examined in that area of the body. And if your family, friends, boss, and even your doctor are not particularly sympathetic, is it surprising that you may get anxious, depressed, moody, and yes, maybe even neurotic or obsessive about it?

*Take comfort!* There is a great deal you can do to help yourself. By the time you have finished this book, you will have a good idea how you can keep your irritable bowel very much under control.

## What Are They Talking About?— A Glossary of Terms

You've waited three months for an appointment to see the specialist; now you've waited for an hour in the "waiting room." At last, someone calls you:

"Mrs. Jones, Room 7, please." In Room 7 are two doctors and a nurse.

"Good morning, come in. It's Mrs. Jones, isn't it? What's your problem? Yes, yes, yes, I see, I see."

From then on you might as well not be there. Words and phrases you've never heard before are tossed around from one doctor to the other: *postprandial pain* (Does that mean pain in my tummy?), *rectal dissatisfaction* (I'm not particularly dissatisfied), *irritable bowel* (Me? irritable?), *motility, intestinal transit,* and so on. Then the doctor says, "We'll do a *sigmoidoscopy* (A what?) and a *barium enema* (I don't like the sound of that)."

"Thank you, Mrs. Jones. We'll arrange some tests for you. Goodbye—next, please."

Well, what was all that about? They were talking about you, but did you understand what they were saying?

So many of us wait passively for them to do things to us—they make appointments for us, they ask the questions, they do the tests, they carry out the treatment.

But it's your body. You've lived with it all your life—you've fed it, washed it, clothed it, exercised it, cared for it. The more you understand how it works, what it can do for you, why it goes wrong and, most important, how you can help put it right, the more you will be in control of your own health.

This chapter will help you to understand what is going on with your bowels, in the belief that by understanding your own body you have a much greater chance of making yourself well.

This chapter is about the many words and phrases you may hear doctors use in reference to Irritable Bowel Syndrome. If the words wash over your head, you are not in a position to help your own recovery; if you understand what they mean, you are halfway there. You can also use the glossary on the following pages to look up the meaning of unfamiliar words you may encounter in other chapters of this book.

# Glossary

*Abdominal:* anything to do with the abdomen or stomach

*Abdominal distension:* your stomach feels or looks bloated and full

*Antispasmodic:* a drug used to reduce spasm and to loosen tight muscles

*Anal spasm:* when the muscle of the anus goes into sudden contraction, usually painful

*Anus:* the circular band of muscle at the lower end of the rectum

*Barium enema:* a test that gives an x-ray picture of your entire colon using liquid barium (See Chapter 2)

*Bowel:* the area you may vaguely think of as your "guts"; it consists of the small intestine (which is about 25 feet long) and the large intestine (which is about 5 feet long) and spans the area from the bottom of your ribs downwards (See page 22)

*Bulking agents:* usually a form of fiber with a psyllium-based or synthetic agent (such as Metamucil or Fiberall) or given to bulk out the stools and make them soft and easier to pass

*Call to stool:* the urge to have a bowel movement

*Colic:* severe pain in the abdomen, caused by spasm of the muscles

*Colon:* the main part of the large intestine (See page 22)

*Constipation:* straining to pass stools or passing stools less than every three days

*Defecation:* the act of emptying the bowels of waste material; having a bowel movement

*Diarrhea:* passing frequent watery or loose bowel movements

*Dyspareunia:* pain during sexual intercourse

*Enzyme:* a substance that aids digestion by breaking down food into a form that can be used by the body (Some people with IBS do not produce enough of the enzyme lactase, which breaks down the sugars in dairy products.)

*Familial:* anything that runs in the family

*Feces:* the waste that you pass when you have a bowel movement; also known as stools

*Flatulence:* feeling full of gas; passing lots of gas

*Flatus:* the gas that builds up in your gut

*Fiber:* substance found in the cellular walls of plants that is not absorbed and digested by the human gut

*Functional:* a condition that has no known physical cause and so is assumed to be caused by the personality or the environment

*Gastrointestinal:* concerning the part of your body that deals with the digestion of food

*Idiopathic:* used to describe a condition that has no apparent cause

*Intermittent pain:* a pain that is not constant but occurs from time to time

*Intestinal transit:* the movement of food through your digestive system

*Intolerance (to food):* certain foods disagree with you and possibly make your IBS worse

*Lactase:* an enzyme that breaks down lactose during digestion; some people with IBS do not have enough of this enzyme in their bodies and cannot digest dairy products properly

*Lactose:* a sugar that occurs naturally in milk and can aggravate IBS in some people

*Laxative:* something you take to stop constipation

*Micturition:* the act of emptying the bladder; passing urine

*Motility:* the contractions of the intestine or colon

*Mucus:* a slimy substance, sometimes passed with a bowel movement or even by itself

*Nausea:* a feeling of being sick to your stomach

*Organic disease:* something wrong with one or more of your internal organs; many IBS sufferers fear they have an organic disease such as cancer or ulcerative colitis, but IBS is more a problem concerning the functioning of the digestive system

*Overreactive:* the term applied to a bowel that reacts more than normal to certain foods, distension, stress, and other stimuli

*Physiological:* having to do with the normal functioning of the body

*Postprandial pain:* a pain, usually in the stomach, that comes on after meals

*Prognosis:* the doctor's thoughts on how the condition will progress, how long it will last, and what will happen next

*Purgative:* an agent that cleanses the bowel; a laxative

*Rectal dissatisfaction:* the feeling after completing a bowel movement that there is still more stool to come

*Rectum:* the last part of the large intestine, where waste matter is stored before finally being passed out of your body through the anus

*Refractory:* used to describe something that doesn't respond well to treatment

*Sigmoidoscopy:* a test that checks your lower colon by insertion of a flexible tube into your anus (See Chapter 2)

*Spasm:* sudden contraction of the muscles; doctors often prescribe antispasmodic drugs because much of the pain of IBS is due to muscles being in spasm, with pain coming in waves

*Spastic:* being in a state of spasm

*Syndrome:* a collection of symptoms

*Transit:* the speed with which food passes through your system, from the time you put it in your mouth until you pass it out as a bowel movement

*Urinary frequency:* needing to empty the bladder often

*Vomiting:* throwing up; regurgitating

Now that you understand the meaning of the words doctors may use about Irritable Bowel Syndrome, you may be interested to know more about the area of your body that all this applies to—the digestive system. This is described in the next section.

## The Digestive System— A Layperson's Guide to IBS

The food you eat is not much use to your body in the form of roast beef, fish and chips, lentils, apples, bread, yogurt, or anything else you put in your mouth. For all these complicated things to be useful, they must be broken down into simple substances that your body can assimilate. This is the process of *digestion.* Proteins become amino acids, which build muscles, hair, nails, skin, kidneys, liver cells, and bone marrow. Fats are absorbed and stored as a source of future energy. They also provide body fat for warmth and for protection of the bones and organs. Carbohydrates become sugars to provide energy for instant use. Vitamins and minerals are absorbed into the bloodstream, and are important in maintaining good health.

In the process of digestion, food travels along about 30 feet of tubing in which it is ground up, churned about, broken down, acted upon by chemicals, and dehydrated (has water drawn from it). It finally leaves your body a day or two later. (See the diagram on page 23.)

When you put food in your mouth, your teeth cut and grind it. Saliva helps the teeth to break down the food and makes the food slippery so that it can slide down the *esophagus* (or gullet). The food is then squeezed down the esophagus by *peristalsis*, a process involving alternating waves of muscular relaxation and contraction. Peristalsis occurs at most stages of digestion, including in the bowel, as we will see later.

From the esophagus the food enters the stomach. To most people's surprise, the stomach is not in the middle of the abdomen but behind the ribs. It is a muscular bag that prepares food for absorption into the bloodstream; in it the food is churned around like in a food mixer for about two to four hours. After enzymes and acids have worked on the food, it leaves the stomach looking rather like a thick soup.

The rest of the digestive process takes place in about 30 feet of tubing called the *bowel*, which is of interest to you if you have IBS.

The first 20 feet or so of the bowel is the *small intestine*—called "small" because the tube is a little over one inch in diameter. It is coiled in the central part of the abdomen, approximately behind the umbilicus (belly button). For several hours, digestive juices act on the food until it is liquid enough to be absorbed through the walls of the small intestine and into the bloodstream, where nutrients can be carried throughout the body, to be used for building and repairing.

For the food that's still left, the next stop is the *large intestine*, also known as the *colon*. The changeover point between small and large intestine is low down on the right-hand side of your abdomen which is where the small intestine ends and the large intestine starts. The large intestine is about two-and-a-half inches wide and about five feet long, and wrinkled like a concertina. It passes up the right hand side, across the middle of your abdomen about level with your belly button, and down the left hand side. This is the direction that the food travels in the large intestine, taking about one to three days. Here the last stages of digestion are completed, as water from the semiliquid mass is absorbed back into the body, and the waste material that is left is stored temporarily until there is enough for it to be eliminated from the body.

By the time the mass reaches the end of the large intestine and enters the rectum at the bottom left hand side of the abdomen, it is quite compact, fairly dry, and brown. Glands produce mucus, which forms a protective coating for the feces and makes it easier for the feces to pass out of the anus. The anus is a strong band of muscle that opens to allow waste material to leave and then closes tightly afterward.

Food is moved along the large intestine by peristalsis. These waves are stimulated by three conditions:

1. By a large volume of waste material being present inside you

2. By filling the stomach with another meal, which causes signals to be sent to the brain to open the bowels and make room for the next lot

3. By getting exercise

The nature of peristalsis causes some of the symptoms of IBS and will be discussed in greater detail later on.

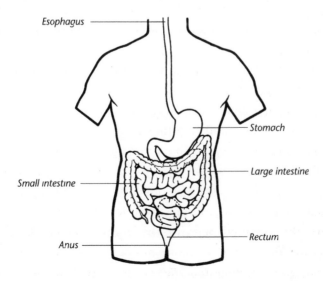

# 2

# Symptoms of IBS

## Medical Investigations and Treatments

> It is a good rule of thumb that if many treatments are in use for the same disease, it is because there is no real treatment known for that disease.
>
> —Peter Parish, *Medicines: A Guide for Everybody*

In the past, indeed until quite recently, people with IBS had appendix removals, intensive abdominal investigations, major gynecological operations, numerous x-rays, and prescriptions for a whole range of pills and potions to rid them of the strange collection of symptoms we now recognize as Irritable Bowel Syndrome. Not surprisingly, these drastic measures were not usually very successful since doctors were seldom treating the real cause of the problem. Luckily, things are different now.

The first thing your doctor will want to do is make sure that what you have really is IBS and not something else. Having done that, she will recommend treatment.

Even if you decide that you want to treat your condition yourself, or you want to receive treatment from a practitioner of alternative medicine, it really is most important that first of all you get a correct diagnosis from a qualified doctor. That way, you can be sure that you are treating the right thing and that nothing serious is being overlooked.

The first part of this chapter discusses the more typical examinations you may have. They may take place in your doctor's office or in a hospital outpatient department. It is unlikely you would have to stay in the hospital as an inpatient. If you are under about 40, the doctor may feel confident to make a diagnosis solely on the basis of your medical history and a brief physical examination alone, without arranging any tests. The second part of the chapter discusses the drugs and other treatments the doctor may recommend, having reached a diagnosis.

First, the doctor will ask you a series of questions. Your answers to the questions will often enable the doctor to decide whether you have IBS without the need to subject you to lots of tests.

You will probably be asked

—When did you first start getting these symptoms?

—Did anything specific trigger them?

—How often do they occur?

—Where exactly is the pain?

—Have you had diarrhea and/or constipation before?

—Do your bowel habits change?

—Have they recently changed?

—Have you lost weight recently?

—Does your stomach look or feel bloated or distended?

—Do you pass mucus with a bowel movement or even on its own?

—Have you ever had bleeding from the anus?

—Have you recently had a bout of gastroenteritis ("holiday tummy")?

—Did you get stomach aches as a child?

—Do any of your family have these symptoms?

—Do the symptoms become worse when you are tense, anxious, or under stress? Or when you eat particular foods?

—Can you do anything to make the symptoms better or worse?

—Do you or your family have an intolerance to dairy products or to wheat products? How much of these do you eat?

Depending on the answers and on your age, your doctor may suggest some physical tests. She may do some of them herself or refer you to a specialist. If you are under 40, she may want to check for a peptic ulcer, for gall bladder disease, ulcerative colitis, and Crohn's disease. If you are over 40, she will also want to be sure there is no sign of malignancy (cancer) in the bowel. If you had an abusive childhood your intestinal nervous system may be hyper-reactive. Specialized x-rays called PET scans have shown differences that exist in the brain of patients with ibs.

Because of the nature of IBS, it is not at present possible to do a single test that definitively confirms Irritable Bowel Syndrome. So, in some cases the doctor will want to do one or two investigations to rule out the diseases that IBS mimics before a firm conclusion can be made. Symptoms in patients with lactose intolerance or intolerance to wheat protein (celiac disease) are exacerbated by the visceral hypersensitivity present in IBS.

The first test will almost certainly be a *rectal examination*. The doctor will probably ask you to take off your clothes below the waist, lie on the examination table on your left side, and bend your legs up slightly. After putting on thin rubber gloves, the doctor will insert one finger into the rectum and feel around inside. This simple test will be able to tell the condition of your rectum. It will probably be a bit uncomfortable, and you may feel embarrassed, but don't forget that the doctor does this kind of thing every day.

Good doctors will recognize your embarrassment and will do all they can to put you at ease.

Other likely investigations for IBS are blood tests, a sigmoid-oscopy, and a barium enema.

Most people have had *blood tests* from time to time. A small area of skin, usually in the arm, is cleaned with an alcohol swab. A fine needle is inserted into a vein, and a small quantity of blood is drawn out into a syringe. The blood sample will be checked for generalized infection, anemia, and the condition of the liver and kidneys. If you predominantly have constipation, it will be important for the physician to measure the transit of material through your colon. This can be done by following the expulsion of radio-opaque markers from the colon. A delay in evacuation can be from a poorly propulsive colon or from an outlet obstruction caused by a dysfunctional pelvic floor.

A *sigmoidoscopy* is an examination to test for disease in the rectum and lower colon. You will need to have an almost empty digestive system for a sigmoidoscopy to be successful, so you will be asked not to eat anything for 24 hours beforehand. You will be asked to lie in the same position as for the rectal examination. The doctor will insert into the rectum one end of an instrument called a flexible sigmoidoscope, which is a very flexible tube one-half inch in diameter and about 24 inches long, with a light at the end. By shining the light into the rectum the doctor will be able to see clearly the condition of the rectum and the lower end of the colon. Any growths (cancerous or noncancerous) will be visible, as will any other abnormal condition such as inflammation. This examination, as you can imagine, can be quite uncomfortable and for some people may be rather painful. But most people who have it feel reassured that the whole area has been thoroughly examined. If, having looked, the doctor says that you do not have any inflammation or cancer of the rectum, you will probably feel greatly relieved.

A sigmoidoscopy has one other benefit: the process of insert-
ing the tube into the rectum causes the rectum to become distended and often reproduces exactly the kind of pain you get with
IBS. Many people are reassured to make the connection between
a distended rectum and the pain of IBS and therefore are more
motivated to take steps to avoid constipation.

A *barium enema* helps to check for organic disease of the whole
colon and can also provide evidence of an irritable colon. You will
need to have an almost empty digestive system for a barium enema
to be successful, so you will be asked not to eat anything for several hours beforehand. You will be taken to the x-ray department,
where a tube will be inserted into the rectum, and a small quantity of thick white liquid will pass through the tube. This procedure
may be carried out on a table that allows you to be tilted slightly in
different positions, so that the liquid can reach every part of the
bowel. The tube is then withdrawn. The white liquid will show up
brightly on the x-ray, and any problems or irregularities over the
entire length of the large intestine will be clearly visible. If you
have a spastic or irritable colon, this will also show up. After the x-
ray, you will eliminate the white liquid as if it were a very runny and
gassy bowel movement.

Some hospitals have a slightly different procedure: you will be
asked to eat nothing after midnight and to take a laxative at bedtime. Next day you may have a simple x-ray of the abdominal area,
and after that undergo the same procedure for filling up the intestine with the thick white liquid. Your intestines are then x-rayed.
You may then be asked to empty your bowel for the whole area to
be x-rayed again.

If diarrhea is your main symptom, you may also have tests for
lactose intolerance and possibly a biopsy of the small intestine. For
the biopsy, you swallow a small metal capsule attached to a suction
tube. When the capsule reaches the right part of the bowel, the
doctor will apply suction to the tube, and a tiny piece from the wall

of the bowel will be sucked into the capsule and removed for examination.

Just a word here about attitudes people have to tests in general. Most people are pleased to have tests to get reassurance that they have nothing seriously wrong with them; when the results are normal, they consider that the end of the matter. However, there is a small group of people who like having tests, who like having a hospital appointment to keep, who even like having operations. Are you one of these? If so, recognize it in yourself and realize that this behavior may cause you to receive less sympathy than you feel you deserve from your doctor, your family, and your friends.

In the past (and unfortunately even now occasionally), many doctors would say something like, "We have done tests, and there is nothing wrong with you," and leave it at that. If you still complained of stomach pain or changing bowel habits or a distended tummy, the doctor would probably dismiss you as a hypochondriac, prescribe tranquilizers, and hope you would go away. After all, tests prove that there is nothing wrong with you.

Today, particularly if your doctor is kind and caring, she may say, "We will do some tests just to check that you haven't got disease A, B, or C, and I expect the tests will be normal." So, when they are normal, this is just what you and she expect. And she will probably explain that you have Irritable Bowel Syndrome and will outline what it is, what it is not, how she can help you, and also how you can help yourself.

IBS cannot be helped by having an operation, but there are several types of drugs that are very effective. The most common are

—*Antispasmodics* to make the bowel muscle relax and to relieve the colicky spasm that causes so much pain. They appear to have no serious side effects, though they may impair driving ability or affect your blood pressure.

—*Bulk-forming agents*, usually based on fiber. These make the stools soft, bulky, and easy to pass. They, too, appear to have no side effects. There are natural fibers, like psyllium, that may be broken down by bacteria into gases. Synthetic fibers such as polycarbophil are more inert.

—*Antidepressants.* Originally prescribed for the depression that affects many IBS sufferers, some of these drugs also work directly to relieve abdominal pain and dampen the activity of neurons that send signals back and forth between the gut and the brain. Recent research confirms that these medications can be helpful even where depression isn't a problem. Since antidepressants must be used continually to be effective, they are generally only prescribed for the most drastic, chronic cases of IBS. Also, they often have side effects, and it is not in your best interest to continue the long-term use of drugs that affect your mind. Some drugs in the antidepressant class (such as low-dose tricyclics) may decrease the hypersensitivity of the sensory nervous system in IBS.

—*Motility drugs.* Many advances have been made in developing drugs that alter the motility or mucosal function in the bowel. The serotonin type 4 agonist tegaserod (Zelnorm) can stimulate the colon and also decrease pain from IBS. This drug is useful in patients with constipation. The serotonin type 3 antagonist, alosetron (lotronex) decreases both diarrhea and pain. Lubiprostone (amitiza) activates a special channel in the muscosa of the colon, increases the fluid in the stool, and improves bowel function.

—*Experimental drugs*, including a drug that blocks the brain's receptors for one form of seratonin. Seratonin is a neurotransmitter, a chemical substance that carries signals from all parts of the body to the brain. Among other things, this neurotransmitter is responsible for our perception of pain; the drug may help dull the perception of intestinal pain, which would benefit those IBS sufferers who are especially sensitive to pain in the gut. Another drug being tested by medical researchers is fedotozine, which numbs sensory nerves.

Where gas is a problem, peppermint oil capsules are often effective. You can obtain much the same effect yourself by sipping a few drops of peppermint essence in a small glass of warm water, or by sucking sweets containing oil of peppermint.

For diarrhea, you may be prescribed substances such as Lomotil, diphenoxylate, or loperamide.

For constipation, the most effective drugs are the bulk-forming agents, though you will probably be advised to eat more fiber in your diet. Don't be tempted to take laxatives that you buy over the counter. Unless used extremely rarely, they can make IBS worse.

For other ways to reduce stomach pain, see the next section.

The types of drugs mentioned previously are usually quite effective, particularly over a short period. But since IBS is often a long-term condition, drugs alone cannot solve the problem permanently. If you can accept that what you eat, how you live, and how you view life will probably heal your bowel more effectively than anything else, you are already half-way along the road to recovery.

If you must take drugs, you should plan to do so for as short a time as possible. Once the bulk laxatives have given you a soft, unformed bowel movement every day for two weeks, see if you can make this happen by diet alone. For most people, this should be possible.

When you are confident that the antispasmodics have reduced your stomach pain, take a fresh look at the tension in you that is causing your bowel muscles to seize up. Then you will become less dependent on drugs. After all, if you see drugs as the only way of getting relief, you may feel a sense of helplessness and dependence on them. When you realize you can improve your condition for yourself, this will lift your spirits and help you take control of your own health.

You will find many ideas on how you can help yourself in this book. There is no suggestion, however, that you will find a permanent lifelong cure, because for many people this just will not happen. The longer you have had IBS, the harder it is to be rid of it completely. But there is no doubt at all that by handling it properly, you should be able to live more peacefully with it.

Once your IBS has been diagnosed and treatment (conventional or alternative) started, you will most likely not need to visit your doctor as often as you might have done before. But there are other causes of abdominal pain, and even IBS sufferers can get appendicitis, peptic ulcers, and heart trouble. Also, although IBS doesn't cause cancer, it doesn't prevent it either. So there are a few symptoms that, if they should occur, you must not ignore:

Blood in the stools or urine

Vomiting blood

Very severe abdominal pain

Indigestion-type pain that persists for more than a day or two

Excessive thirst

Unexplained loss of weight or appetite

Unexplained change in bowel habits that lasts for a month or more and causes disruption to your life

Unexplained increase in the size of your stomach

IBS symptoms that change or get noticeably worse

If you get any of these, see your doctor as soon as possible.

## Do You Have Abdominal Pain?

Pain in the gut is what drives most people with an irritable bowel to the doctor. This pain is generally down on the lower left-hand side of the abdomen, but it could also be in the center or on the right. It may range from a dull ache to pain of such severity that the sufferer doubles up and even sometimes goes to a hospital emergency room. The pain may last from a few minutes to many hours and may be spasmodic or persistent. Once again, there are so many symptoms that it's not surprising it has taken so long for doctors to piece them all together into one recognizable condition.

The pain of IBS is generally colicky, cramplike, and spasmodic. The spasm may affect the whole bowel or just one section, so the position and intensity of the pain may vary. People with IBS will typically describe the pain as "sharp," "stabbing," "knifelike," "burning," "cutting," or "very strong." Some find the pain comes on after meals; those with diarrhea often find the pain comes on with the bowel movement and then gets better; those with constipation usually find that the pain only goes away when they stop being constipated. When the colon is distended (enlarged and stretched), this can produce pain in some unlikely parts of the body: the back, shoulders, thigh, and genitals. In contrast with this, some people with IBS find they get very little pain, just the other main symptoms.

This section suggests ways of coping with abdominal pain. First, get it checked by the doctor. It is important to be sure your pain is due to IBS and not something else. Once you have your diagnosis, try these various ideas, and see which works best for you:

—Take antispasmodic drugs, as prescribed by the doctor.

—Take homeopathic nux vomica 6 or 30. Take two tablets one night, two the following morning, and two the following night, then stop. You should notice an improvement in two to four weeks; if your IBS recurs later, repeat this dose. (Homeopathy is discussed on pages 152–55.)

—When the pain strikes you, breathe deeply, concentrating on the passage of air in your nostrils and focusing your attention on a point between your eyebrows at the top of your nose. Exhale slowly. Try to keep your abdominal muscles relaxed the whole time—do not tense them up.

—Lie flat, perhaps with your arms over your head if this feels comfortable, with a hot water bottle on your tummy. You may also find it helpful to use an electric blanket, though you should take great care when doing so.

—Lie on your back on the floor, head supported by a soft object, knees drawn up, and feet flat on the floor.

—Use a hot compress. Take a small towel, wring it out in hot water, fold it to a convenient size, and leave it on your abdomen until it cools.

—Do something active—do some gentle stretching exercises or go for a walk. If you are in bed or in a chair, get up and walk around vigorously.

—Get rid of the constipation that might be the cause of the stomach pain.

—Do something to take your mind off the pain. If you have ever attended prenatal classes, practice the labor-pain exercises you learned. Otherwise, do something—anything—that requires concentration and makes you think of something else.

—Avoid antacid indigestion tablets. Their high-alkaline content destroys the stomach's natural acids, which digest food. If you take these tablets too often, the stomach responds by producing extra acid, which can cause more pain or digestive problems and eventually lead to a gastric ulcer.

—Infuse $1/3$ to $2/3$ ounce of hops (available from home-brewing shops and health food stores) in 1 quart of boiling water for ten minutes and drink a cupful after meals.

—Infuse $1/3$ to $2/3$ ounce of balm or lemon balm in the same way, and drink a cupful with meals.

—Heat a teaspoonful of fennel seeds in a cup of milk and drink it while fairly hot.

—When cooking, use herbs that aid digestion and that tonify and soothe the bowel. These include cumin, fennel, fenugreek, garlic, ginger, goldenseal, marjoram, mint, parsley, pau d'arco, rosehips, rosemary, sage, slippery elm, and thyme.

—Infuse $\frac{1}{6}$ ounce of lavender in a quart of boiling water. Leave for five minutes, strain, and drink three cups a day between meals.

—Infuse four or five leaves of mint (dried or fresh) in a cup of boiling water, leave for five minutes, strain, and drink twice a day after meals. If this causes insomnia, use only two leaves per cup and drink one cupful a day, in the morning. You could also use peppermint essence oil in a glass of warm water.

—Infuse $\frac{2}{3}$ to 1 ounce of fresh or dried thyme in a quart of water for about five minutes. Strain and drink three cupfuls a day after meals.

—Infuse $\frac{1}{3}$ to $\frac{2}{3}$ ounce of chamomile in the same way and drink three cups a day after meals.

—Try a preparation of skullcap or valerian root to calm the nerves that regulate the muscles of the intestine.

Most of these ingredients should be available from health food stores or large supermarkets.

The following homeopathic remedies may help cramping pains:

—*Belladonna:* if you feel distended but better when doubled up

—*Bryonia:* if you feel better when lying still and worse from heat

—*Colocynth:* if you can't keep still and feel better doubled up

—*Magnesia phosphorica:* if applying heat to your abdomen makes you feel better

If the pain is caused by *gas*, try the following ideas:

—Take steps to avoid constipation. A blocked rectum prevents gas from escaping, so it has no alternative but to build up in your intestines and cause discomfort. By keeping your rectum relatively empty, you allow that gas to escape.

—When gas builds up, sit up straight or stand up straight and, if possible, walk around vigorously.

—You may find a low-fiber diet helpful: more peeled vegetables; fish; lean meat; white rice, bread, and pasta; and less whole wheat bread or pasta, cereals, and dried fruit.

—Be aware that you may be swallowing excess air as you eat or drink—try to avoid doing this.

—Infuse a cut root of angelica in boiling water for several minutes, strain, and drink a small glassful before meals.

—Chew raw angelica root or leaves.

—Chew mustard seeds with plenty of water.

—Put a few drops of peppermint oil in warm water and sip.

—Suck on sweets containing real oil of peppermint.

—Chew charcoal tablets.

—Add a teaspoon of cinnamon or nutmeg to warm milk, then sweeten with honey and drink.

—Infuse any of the following in boiling water for about ten minutes, and drink when it has cooled slightly (you may prefer the drink sweetened with honey): fresh or dried basil leaves, grated ginger root, half a fresh lemon, or some marjoram.

And finally, some exercises for *general improvement of the abdomen:*

—This exercise strengthens all the abdominal muscles with a minimum of strain. Lie on your back with knees bent, feet flat on the floor. Clasp your hands behind your head, resting your head on your hands. Gently begin to sit up, without putting strain on your neck, raising yourself two to three inches until your shoulder blades are just off the floor. Hold this position for five seconds or longer. Breathe deeply. Repeat exercise several times. Listen to your body—when your muscles ache, it's time to stop.

—Lie on your back with your knees bent and your feet flat on the floor close to your buttocks. Lift your hips off the floor, drawing the abdominal muscles up and in at the same time. Then lower your hips. Repeat several times; stop when you feel tired.

—Stand with legs apart, knees bent, hands pressing on thighs. As you breathe in, pull your abdominal muscles in and up, hold your breath, and pump your belly in and out using your muscles. Stop pumping when you need to breathe out, take a normal breath, then breathe in and repeat. Aim to do 10 to 15 pumpings at a time.

—Self-massage of the colon: lie on your back on a flat surface, and roll a tennis ball firmly up the right side of the abdomen, across the bottom of the rib cage, and down the left-hand side (that is, in the direction the digested food travels). This exercise is particularly effective if you do it first thing in the morning before rising.

—Cup one hand with fingers and thumbs closed tightly as if you were holding water in your hand. Then, keeping the hand in this position, gently strike your colon rhythmically with the hollowed hand and fingertips, keeping the wrists as loose as possible, with palm facing downwards. As in the previous exercise, work up the right side of the abdomen, across the middle, and down the left side. Do this exercise lying down.

## Do You Have Constipation?

The symptoms of IBS are much more common in people with long-term constipation than in most other people. In fact, when people who do not have IBS are deliberately made constipated during research experiments, they start to develop some of the usual symptoms of an irritable bowel; and when their constipation is artificially ended by laxatives, their IBS symptoms cease.

Many people with IBS find constipation, either constant or intermittent, is their main symptom. In addition, they will probably have pain in the stomach, because the more constipated a person is, the more likely it is that he or she has abdominal pain.

One of the main causes of IBS is an irregularity in the speed with which food passes through the digestive system—too slowly and you get constipation; too quickly and you get diarrhea.

What is constipation? Most people who get constipation would probably say that the stools are difficult to push out, that even after a bowel movement they have the feeling there is more to come, and that they don't have bowel movements as often as they think they should. Most doctors would agree that constipation is straining to pass the stools, having fewer than three bowel movements a week, and passing small, hard stools.

While most people have about one bowel movement a day, some have one every two or three days, some once a week. As a general rule, if your bowel movements are no more frequent than twice a day and no less frequent than twice a week, that is quite normal, provided that you have a soft, well-formed movement without pain or straining.

Generally, your bowel habits should remain fairly constant throughout your life, changing only when you have a change of environment, such as going on vacation or eating different food. If your bowel pattern remains unchanged, it is unlikely you have any disease of the digestive system. But if you have more constipation or more diarrhea that is not connected with a change in your lifestyle, and the change lasts for several weeks, it might be a good idea to see your doctor.

People with IBS often describe their bowel movement as "like rabbit pellets," or "small, lumpy stool," or "stringy," or "hard and dry." Let's look at why this happens.

In the normal colon, feces are propelled along by peristalsis, in much the same way as food is propelled down the esophagus toward the stomach. (Remind yourself of your digestive system by looking at the diagram on page 23.) The muscle walls of the colon work best when they are propelling feces that are soft and bulky; this keeps the muscle walls a regular distance apart (remember, the colon is a tube). If the feces are small and hard, the colon must squeeze in further than its muscular walls can comfortably manage. This causes pressure to build up and muscles to go into spasm in the colon, which causes pain.

When the muscle is in spasm, it no longer propels the feces in smooth waves toward the rectum. Instead, it just keeps squeezing and relaxing, often causing intense pain. And instead of the feces moving evenly on their way, they become compressed and divided into tiny segments with each squeeze, causing the typical hard, pelletlike stools of IBS.

Many people remain constipated for years. As a result, they are more likely to get diverticulosis, piles (hemorrhoids), and varicose veins. They may also have lower back pain or stomach ache from a rectum that is always too full with hard, compacted feces, not to mention extra problems such as headaches, lethargy, loss of appetite, and a general feeling of being "under the weather."

In addition, because food remains so much longer than normal in the digestive system, there is more chance for bacteria to build up allowing harmful materials to be absorbed into the bloodstream. With most people, food remains in the gut for about one-and-a-half to two-and-a-half days; for those who are constipated, food remains for an average of five days and may even last up to ten. Although unusual, some people with IBS can go a month without a bowel movement.

What causes constipation? As with most conditions, there are many causes. The most common are

—Lack of exercise

—Not enough dietary fiber in the diet

—Ignoring the call to empty the bowel

—Taking certain drugs

—Certain medical conditions

Many drugs cause constipation, so if you are taking any of the following and constipation is a problem to you, talk to your doctor about it:

—Pain killers (particularly the strong ones)

—Anticonvulsants (used in epilepsy and similar conditions)

—Water-reducing drugs (for heart conditions)

—Iron tablets

—Drugs for high blood pressure

Antacid tablets can also cause constipation, leading to a vicious circle: you have a pain in your stomach, so you take antacid tablets, so you may become more constipated, so you get more stomach pain.

Lastly, one of the main causes of constipation is, ironically, overuse of laxatives. (See pages 45–48.)

If constipation is your problem, here is what you can do about it. The rules are quite simple, and for most people they will do the trick.

—The most natural treatment for simple constipation is a high- fiber diet. (Read Chapter 6 for more on this.)

—Drink plenty of fluids, preferably nonalcoholic and some-times warmed. Tannin in black teas tends to constipate, so drink herb tea instead. There are some delicious ones available; if you find them a bit sharp, try adding honey.

—Drink at least 64 ounces of water a day.

—Some foods may make your IBS worse. If you suspect this may be so, try the simple diet on page 190 in order to identify which foods these may be.

—When you eat, a "food-now-entering-stomach" message is sent to the brain. Then the brain sends a message to the intestines saying "make room for an incoming meal." This message causes the large intestine to empty its contents into the storage depot of the rectum. So try to empty the bowel just after meals, when your body is preparing to move each batch of food along to the next stage. This sys-tem works most effectively after the first meal of the day, so be particularly aware of it after breakfast.

—Try to have your bowel movements at the same time each day.

—Allow plenty of time for each bowel movement. Try get-ting up twenty minutes earlier in the morning, eat a leisurely breakfast, then disappear to the toilet with a book, magazine, or newspaper for at least 10 to 15 min-utes. Don't push or strain, as this could cause piles (hem-orrhoids); just allow time for the rectum to empty out.

—An early morning train, bus, or car journey may inhibit the natural morning urge to empty the bowels. So either fit in time for a long visit to the toilet before your morn-ing journey or allow time for it when you arrive. A hot drink either before or during the journey may help to get your insides moving.

—Never neglect the urge to "go." When the rectum is comfortably full, the stools are covered with slimy mucus to make them easier to pass. But if the stools remain too long in the rectum, this mucus is absorbed back into the body, making the stools hard, dry, and painful to pass. So when your body says "go," go! That way you work with your body, not against it.

—Since exercise is one of the things that triggers the bowel to empty, get plenty of it. This gives your brain a chance to send "exercise" messages to the bowel. It needn't be wildly energetic; a brisk walk every day is fine for most people. Exercise also improves your capacity to withstand stress and keeps your internal muscles in good condition. Many digestive ailments are caused because muscles in the abdomen are too slack, so they sag, and the contents of the abdomen are compressed downward. This produces congestion, sluggish bowel movements, and constipation.

Here are some traditional remedies for constipation:

—Infuse $1/10$ to $1/5$ ounce of basil leaves or flower tips in boiling water. Strain and drink. Basil also has antispasmodic properties.

—Eat a raw apple in its skin for breakfast every day.

—Psyllium seed, with a full glass of water, keeps the stool soft.

—Drink barley juice or wheatgrass.

—Simmer two pounds of carrots in four cups of water for about one to two hours. Blend in a blender. Take as a soup.

—Soak figs or prunes overnight in water. The figs can be eaten uncooked, but prunes should be cooked before eating. Drink the water they have been cooked in, too.

—Eat kiwi fruit (a traditional remedy from New Zealand) from time to time.

—Eat charcoal biscuits (obtainable from pharmacists or health food stores).

—Drink a ½ cup of aloe vera juice in the morning and evening.

—Take natural licorice, as sweets or in stick form.

—Massage your lower back with a blend of essential oils: 20 drops of marjoram plus five drops of rose in two fluid ounces of vegetable oil. Essential oils can be obtained from many health food stores.

## Do You Have Diarrhea?

As you will know by now, diarrhea is one of the main symptoms of IBS. You may have it on its own, or alternating with constipation, or with or without mucus. The usual pattern is to have a period of constipation with the typical "rabbit pellets," then out it all comes as a rather explosive diarrhea.

In fact, this is not typical diarrhea. *Typical* or *infective diarrhea*—also known as gastroenteritis—is usually caused by an infection or by contaminated food or water. As the body tries to get rid of whatever has contaminated it, the typical symptoms occur: upset stomach, vomiting, abdominal pain, and great quantities of very loose stools. You will probably feel dreadful, all limp and washed out, but when you have gotten rid of whatever made you sick, you will start to feel better again.

The diarrhea of IBS is rather different. The quantity of feces that you pass is much smaller than with infective diarrhea; in fact, over several days it is much the same quantity as an average bowel movement, though more frequent and sloppy. And the looseness is not caused by any infection or contamination.

With the diarrheal form of IBS, you probably get it worse in the morning and feel more settled as the day progresses. The pain may get worse as you have a bowel movement and then disappear. Also, you may have to get up in the night with it. Some people have

IBS and diarrhea without any pain at all. Once again, there are so many variations that it's not surprising it has taken so long to link all the symptoms together.

It is possible that part of your colon does not work as well as it should and passes food on to the rectum before all the water has been properly absorbed, making the stools fairly runny instead of fairly dry. Also, your own rectum may not like being even half-full and may send "emptying" messages too early.

Also, bear in mind that quite a large number of those with the diarrheal form of IBS use laxatives regularly and surreptitiously, and this is probably one of the causes of the problem.

Researchers have discovered that 50 to 60 percent of individuals with the diarrheal form of IBS have an intolerance to one or more foods. You may be one of these if you experience one of the following conditions:

—You have diarrhea as your main symptom.

—You wake up at night needing to have a bowel movement.

—You started to get IBS after an attack of gastroenteritis or a long course of antibiotics.

—You feel very tired or weary.

—You get headaches.

Whether diet is or is not an important cause of your IBS, if you have the diarrheal form of the condition, you most likely have more anxiety than those with the constipation form. After all, you know from those butterflies in your tummy before an important event what the link is between diarrhea and anxiety. So take positive steps to reduce stress and anxiety as a means of helping your irritable bowel. A later chapter on managing stress contains lots of ideas.

Here are some other well-tried remedies for diarrhea:

—Strange as it may seem, the same high-fiber/low-fat diet that is recommended for constipation also works for diarrhea in many people. Bran may work for you, although it may make the stools sticky for a few weeks.

—Bulk fiber supplements (such as Metamucil, Citrucel, or Fiberall) help bind loose stools together.

—Antidiarrheal drugs prescribed by the doctor can be of great benefit, particularly if you get so agitated about being far from the toilet that your whole life is seriously restricted.

—Several herbs help: chamomile, slippery elm bark, blackberry root bark, and pau d'arco are beneficial. Use them in tea form. Ginger tea aids with stomach cramps and pain.

—Mix two teaspoonfuls of cider vinegar in a glass of water and drink before each meal.

—Before any event that is worrying you, try this: add one teaspoonful of honey to one fluid ounce of hot water and stir until the honey melts. Then add two or three drops of essential oil of geranium (obtainable from health food stores) and sip slowly.

—Mix two heaping teaspoonfuls of arrowroot (obtainable from health food stores and pharmacies) with a small quantity of cold water until smooth. Top up with about one pint of boiling water and drink when cool. You may prefer it flavored, with black currant juice for example.

## Beware of Laxatives

Many people use larger and larger quantities of ever-stronger laxatives more and more often, to less and less effect. They are afraid to stop in case they get more constipated; yet one of the main reasons for constipation is overuse of laxatives.

Laxatives are among the most common medicines bought over the counter. In addition, millions of laxatives are prescribed by doctors. Possibly up to 46 percent of the general population use them regularly. This is not only expensive, it is unnecessary and potentially harmful. And you would be surprised how many people with IBS regularly take laxatives and prefer not to tell their doctor.

Laxatives are extensively misused in the mistaken belief that there is some wondrous relationship between good health and a daily emptying of the bowels—"regularity is next to godliness." This just isn't so. It is quite normal to have a bowel movement two or three times a day or two or three times a week. Even going one or two days over what is normal for you is nothing to worry about. As long as your movement is soft, well formed, easy to pass, and the same as it has always been, that's how it should be—you are quite normal.

There really is no known connection between a daily bowel movement and good health. Nor does a less regular bowel-movement pattern indicate poor health, unless the change in pattern is recent, persists for several weeks, or has a noticeable effect on your life.

When you read advertisements for laxatives (whose manufacturers are, after all, trying to sell as much of their product as possible), it is easy to get the impression that missing a bowel movement is something really serious. So you become worried and take a laxative. This empties the whole of the large intestine, and several days pass before a normal quantity of stool forms again. In the meantime, you don't have another bowel movement because there's nothing in the bowel to pass, so you think you are constipated, and you take laxatives again. Thus you never give your body a chance to work normally. If this pattern continues, eventually the bowel muscle becomes damaged and won't work at all, unless there is a laxative to force it into action.

Ideally, the rectum will empty almost completely every day or so, as will about one-third of the contents of the large intestine. To empty everything all at once is not what your body was designed to do.

If you do take laxatives regularly, don't rush to cut down on them. Reduce the dose gradually, perhaps from two doses a day to one dose a day for a few days, then one dose every other day for several days, then two doses a week, then one dose a week, until you can finally stop completely without traumatizing your system.

There are several kinds of laxatives on the market. Some add bulk to the feces to make the bowel muscle propel them more easily; others loosen and lubricate the feces; others stimulate and irritate the bowel. The main types are

—*Bulk-forming laxatives*, usually made from fiber such as psyllium, polycarbophil, or methycellulose (brand names include Metamucil, Fibercon, Fiberall, and Citrucel). These are the ones most commonly prescribed for IBS and are the safest for long-term use. They stimulate the bowel muscles naturally by making the stools moist, soft, bulky, and easier to pass. (They may also help prevent diverticulitis.) Take plenty of fluids with them, as fluid keeps the psyllium soft and prevents it from becoming sticky. (Although the term bulk laxative is one that is still used, it may be a misuse of the word laxative. Fiber supplements do not irritate the bowel, the function of a true laxative in stimulating the bowel. The proper term for these psyllium-based products is bulk-forming agents.) The psyllium-based compounds increase bloating since the cellulose can be broken down by the patient's intestinal bacteria. This reaction occurs less with polycarbophil or methylcellulose.

—*Lubricant laxatives*, such as liquid paraffin. If you take these regularly, your body may fail to absorb some essential vitamins; they can also cause trouble with the bowel wall, liver, and spleen. Liquid paraffin coats some of the food you eat, thus preventing it from being properly digested and absorbed. It also prevents useful bacteria from working, it does not mix with water and so does not soften the feces, and, if you use it regularly, it may leak out through the rectum.

—*Stimulant laxatives*, such as cascara, castor oil, and senna. They increase bowel movements by irritating the lining of the bowel and stimulating the bowel muscles to contract. However, from reading the section on constipation, you now know that it can be very painful if the walls of the bowel contract excessively onto hard, compacted stools. If you have Irritable Bowel Syndrome, it is likely that your colon (or bowel) already contracts at a higher than normal rate, so laxatives of this type will probably make your stomach pain worse. Stimulant laxatives can also be dangerous if, for any reason, you have an obstructed bowel.

—*Saline laxatives*, often called "health salts," make the stools bulkier by causing them to retain water (unlike bulk-forming laxatives, which make stools bulkier by causing them to retain dietary fiber). To do this, saline laxatives may draw fluids from the body and cause it to become dehydrated. They may be harmful to people with kidney disease or who are on diuretics (water-reducing drugs commonly prescribed for heart conditions). If in doubt, ask your doctor whether health salts are a good idea for you.

Finally, don't take laxatives to relieve stomach pains, cramps, or colic. These pains may signal a more serious condition, such as acute appendicitis.

# 3

## Stress and Other Causes of IBS

## What Is Stress?

Stress is normal. It is even desirable (in the right place, at the right time, and in the right quantity). It can add spice to life, that extra something that gives you a buzz and makes you feel stretched, challenged, and stimulated.

In its positive form, stress helps athletes to win, musicians and actors to perform better, artists of all kinds to be more creative, businesspeople to meet deadlines, and all of us to avoid or survive dangerous situations.

Positive stress is when we feel confident we can meet a particular challenge. We feel exhilarated and invigorated by engaging in physical activity, getting the job we wanted, starting a new love affair. Positive emotions—excitement, happiness, confidence, pleasure, laughter, joy, love—increase our ability to withstand stress.

Negative stress isn't necessarily having a heavy work load, or working long hours, or having lots of responsibility and demands made on you, or even having a boring or repetitive job. Negative stress for you is what makes you physically or mentally unwell, those things that your personally find it hard to cope with, those things that get you stewed up inside because of your own attitudes and beliefs.

In the same way that positive emotions increase our ability to withstand stress, so negative emotions reduce this resistance. Emotions such as worry, guilt, anger, hostility, fear, anxiety, boredom, and frustration are fine in small quantities, but if we build up too much of them, we can end up in trouble. When stress first appears, it usually brings with it some physical or mental symptoms (increased heartbeat, excitement, and so on), then we respond to the challenge and cope with the extra demand; so far, so good. But if we have too much in too short a time, or if it goes on for too long, we become overburdened; if, finally, we ignore the warning signs, the final stage is exhaustion, collapse, breakdown, and illness. Does your bowel become more irritable when you are under stress? If so, take comfort—you are not alone.

You may have noticed that one person under stress will develop migraines, another has asthma, others get catarrh, and still others suffer from coronary heart disease, ulcers, skin disorders, or irritable bowel syndrome. It would appear that each of us has a "weak link." Overload it, and it will snap. Most adults and many children find there is one particular part of them that always seems to give way when they are tired, anxious, run down, or under stress of any sort. If you get IBS, then your weak point is probably your gut.

So what is this intangible thing that upsets your insides, that you can't touch, see, or even describe clearly? The more you know about it, the more you will be able to recognize it and then do something about it.

Long ago, our ancestors lived simple lives in caves. They were without the pressures of telephones, daily commutes, traffic jams, high-pressure jobs, and the demands of looking after children while going out to work. The only holdups they met with would be with the greater four-toed mammoth or something similar.

Now just imagine early *Homo sapiens* meeting this mammoth. He would think (in grunts, of course) something like, "This will keep me and the missus in meat and fur for many a moon. I will chase after it. Of course, it may decide I can keep it in meat for a day or so, in which case it will chase after me!" His body would recognize that either of these events would be decidedly stressful and would prepare itself accordingly.

His brain would sends messages to his adrenal glands to produce lots of adrenaline. This would causes vital changes to take place to give him a better chance of survival. The blood would drain from his skin and digestive organs to give more resources to his muscles. Sugars and fats would be released into his blood to provide much-needed energy for all that running. He would breathe faster, so that more oxygen could be made available to burn up the sugar and fat and make it useful quickly. His pupils would enlarge to give him better vision. His blood would thicken so as to coagulate quickly if he were wounded. And his blood pressure would rise as his heart pumped away like crazy, keeping the whole body working in overdrive. He would obviously be very well prepared for fight with the mammoth or for flight away from it.

We have changed a lot in the last few million years. We have moved out of caves, invented computers, landed on the moon, and created designer-label jeans. All very modern. Unfortunately, our bodies have not really kept pace—in evolutionary terms, we are still living in caves.

Like Mr. *Homo sapiens*, whenever we are under stress (whether in a traffic jam, an argument, an extra-hard hour at work, a spell of dreadful boredom, an unhappy marriage, or a job we don't like), we experience the same bodily changes that prepared our ancestor for his fight-or-flight response. Extra adrenaline is produced, and as a result our blood thickens, our digestive system closes down, our heart pumps wildly, our blood pressure rises, fats and sugars release into our body—and then . . . nothing. We are still just where we were five minutes ago. No rushing around, no fighting, no activity to use up all that adrenaline.

What happens, then, to all the physiological changes? Our blood remains thicker for some time, fats and sugars hang around in our bloodstream, our heart takes time to slow down and return to its normal pressure. This is the perfect scenario for coronary heart disease and other stress-related illnesses.

Stress has another effect on our bodies. In addition to producing adrenaline, the adrenal glands help the body fight infection. But constant stress produces changes in these glands that reduce their fighting capacity. That is why, after periods of stress, many people get colds, feel run down and tired, have aches, pains—and digestive disorders. It all has to do with those overloaded adrenal glands. There is also a recognized link between stress and certain types of cancer.

Stress itself does not kill; it's your reaction to it that determines how much it harms you. Some people react strongly to the stress of overwork or of boredom; others to the stress of arguments; others to the stress of a change of diet or to various drugs. How each person reacts depends on previous experiences, personality, culture, and basic genetic susceptibility to stress. In fact, the damage done to your body depends less on the level of stress and much more on your ability to cope with it. Some people cope well, take it all in stride, and genuinely do not seem too bothered by levels of stress that would reduce someone else to a quivering wreck.

So know that in managing stress, there is a great deal you can do to help yourself.

## Are You under Stress?

It's usually not too difficult to see that your spouse, your boss, or your friend is under stress. Likewise, they can probably see what state you are in. But can you?

Why is it, you may ask yourself, that it's all right for other people to be showing signs of stress but not for you? Many people are unwilling to admit to being under stress in case others see them as weak, ineffectual, or unable to cope. They feel that they should be seen as strong and capable, a tower of strength to others, someone to lean on, who can put up with whatever life throws at them and survive unscathed. I hope that by the end of this book you will feel that it's all right to be vulnerable, to give in sometimes, and to have a condition that may be triggered by stress.

Imagine you are quietly living your life when suddenly you get blinding headaches, distorted vision, or severe chest pains. You would take it seriously, go straight to the doctor, submit to tests, take any drugs you are given, and probably make some changes in your way of life to make sure it didn't happen again. But instead, the chances are that your IBS came on gradually—a bit of indigestion, minor abdominal pains, mild food poisoning, nothing to bother about much. So you let it go on and on, not taking it seriously, not making any changes, because the symptoms were not much more than a nuisance.

However, if your IBS is triggered by stress, then ignoring what your body is trying to tell you can make the condition worse, until it becomes quite painful and embarrassing and spoils your enjoyment of life. Symptoms of illness are the body's way of telling you something is wrong. If you develop severe abdominal pain and start vomiting, it could be appendicitis. If you try to cover up the body's warning signs with painkillers or indigestion tablets, you could develop peritonitis, which in extreme cases could be fatal. Emotional symptoms are just as important as physical ones, and ignoring emotional warning signs can be just as serious.

There's no reason to be apologetic or defensive about having a stress-related condition. About half of all people who visit their doctor have some kind of stress-related illness, so you are not at all unusual. But Irritable Bowel Syndrome doesn't exactly make life a laugh-a-minute, and you'd probably be very glad to be rid of it.

## Who Suffers from Stress?

People at any stage of life can experience stress—and IBS:

—Adolescents feel conflicts between the different expectations imposed on them by themselves, their parents, their teachers, and their friends. They want freedom and protection at the same time. Exams, sexual development, disagreements with friends, peer pressure, insecurity, boredom, acne, body image, world issues, the environment . . . all these make adolescence a vulnerable time.

—Young adults may feel pressure from getting married, starting (or not starting) a family, paying mortgages, finding a fulfilling job, and coping with parents' attitudes.

—People "in their prime" (say, from ages 35 to 45) may be "climbing the greasy pole": working long hours, coping with children, taking on responsibility at work, having anxieties about promotions, possibly getting divorced. These are usually the years of maximum financial stretch and the worry that goes with it.

—Those in mid-life crisis may believe "it's now or never." They may fear a job layoff or a long-term illness, the death of their parents or their own pending old age and dependency, their children leaving home and becoming more independent, the continuing need for status, and so on.

All this makes stress a very individual thing. What upsets one person hardly bothers another. But the point here is how you feel or behave when something stressful happens to you. Do you, like someone I'll call Ray, lose your temper, behave in a rude or aggressive way, use obscenities in every sentence, threaten dire consequences to anyone involved, or even use physical violence? Or are you more like someone I'll call Tim—able to remain calm and courteous, talk in a quiet and unthreatening way, make the most of how things are, however annoying, and get on with life without brooding about it all?

Ray is your ideal candidate for something as frightening as a stroke or heart attack. Because he is quite unable to recognize what he finds stressful and even less able to handle it, he probably suffers from some form of stress-related illness, including IBS.

There is also a third character, whom I'll call Penny. Let's say she is stuck in a traffic jam, her hotel room is overbooked, her assistant has phoned in sick, and her computer has broken down. What does she do? She feels just as angry as Ray and yet, unlike Tim, she can't quite take it all in her stride. Inwardly, she is furious with everyone, but she has been brought up to believe it is unlady-like, impolite, and weak to let anyone know how she feels. All her emotions are tightly bottled up inside her; she is frightened of expressing annoyance, disapproval, or anger. Perhaps her father had a violent temper, and she has seen the consequences it had on her mother and the rest of the family; perhaps as a child she was reprimanded for showing her feelings; perhaps her mother put up with whatever life threw at her, and Penny feels she should do the same. Whatever the reason, Penny feels stress just as much as Ray does, and consequently suffers from a stress-related disease.

Whether you find life situations stressful depends on four components:

1. Your basic temperament

2. Your ability to deal with what life throws at you

3. The level of stress you are already under

4. Whether you are a "Type A" personality

You can't do much about 1, but there is quite a bit you can do about the other three. Other things also affect your ability to tolerate stress: your family background, the way you were brought up to handle emotions and to think about different situations, your beliefs and attitudes, and your state of health. In any given situation (from being given a load of work to do in a short time to having an argument with a neighbor), one person may find it stressful, another may find it tolerable, and yet another may even thrive on it. Your life and your digestive system would probably be a lot calmer if you could become more like Tim.

## How Do You Show Signs of Stress?

Stress can show itself in many ways—physically, emotionally, or behaviorally; we all feel stress differently. Although stress-related symptoms are not particularly dramatic, they too have their own signs by which the body is trying to tell you, "There's something wrong here—please do something about it." Look through this list and check off anything that you experience when you feel stressed:

PHYSICAL SIGNS OF STRESS

_____ Tension in your muscles (shoulders, neck, jaw, hands)

_____ Unexplained pains in your back or neck

_____ A knot in your stomach

_____ Nausea (feeling sick to your stomach)

_____ Breathing fast or erratically, or breathlessness

_____ Holding your breath or overbreathing

_____ Headaches or migraines

_____ Indigestion or IBS symptoms

_____ Diarrhea or constipation

_____ General aches and pains

_____ Dry mouth

_____ Menstrual problems

_____ Unusual sweating

_____ Heart palpitations

_____ Feeling restless or jumpy

_____ Sleeping difficulties

EMOTIONAL SIGNS OF STRESS

\_\_\_\_ Depression

\_\_\_\_ Inability to cope

\_\_\_\_ Anxiety or nervousness

\_\_\_\_ Unusual irritability or anger

\_\_\_\_ Irrational fears or feelings of panic

\_\_\_\_ Weepiness

\_\_\_\_ Low self-image

\_\_\_\_ Lack of self-confidence

\_\_\_\_ Feelings of inadequacy

\_\_\_\_ Feelings of hostility or resentment

\_\_\_\_ Aggressiveness

\_\_\_\_ Too much criticism of yourself and others

\_\_\_\_ Feeling like you've "had enough"

\_\_\_\_ Fatigue, apathy, lack of energy

\_\_\_\_ Self-pity

\_\_\_\_ Worry about minor things

\_\_\_\_ Difficulty making rational judgments

\_\_\_\_ Inability to concentrate

\_\_\_\_ Difficulty making simple decisions

\_\_\_\_ Blowing things out of proportion

\_\_\_\_ Inability to communicate about intimate feelings

\_\_\_\_ Hypersensitivity to criticism

BEHAVIORAL SIGNS OF STRESS

\_\_\_\_ Overeating or undereating

____ Insomnia or sleeping too much

____ Drinking or smoking more

____ Being unusually fussy about food

____ Talking much more or less than usual

____ Overworking or avoiding work

____ Losing interest in sex

____ Nail biting

____ Fiddling constantly with your hair

____ Licking your lips frequently

____ Drumming your fingers, jiggling your knees, tapping your feet

____ Driving recklessly

____ Becoming more accident prone

## OTHER SIGNS OF STRESS

As you probably know, stress affects more than just your irritable bowel. It can cause many other complaints and diseases (although most of these can also have other causes):

____ High blood pressure

____ Heart disease

____ Heart attacks

____ Strokes

____ Certain types of cancer

____ Certain types of back pain

____ Tension headaches and migraine

____ Certain types of allergies and asthma

____ Lowered resistance

_____ Duodenal and gastric ulcers

_____ Sexual problems

_____ Hay fever

_____ Rheumatoid arthritis

_____ Diseases of the immune system

_____ Skin conditions, including eczema and acne

_____ Fatigue and lethargy

_____ Alcoholism and drug dependency

_____ Mental illness

_____ Severe depression

As well as medical conditions, stress can also contribute to a whole host of social problems:

_____ Marital breakdowns

_____ Violence

_____ Arguments

_____ Absenteeism at work

Be honest with yourself. You may not like to admit that you lose interest in sex, drive recklessly, lack self-confidence, or blow things out of proportion. But if this is how stress shows itself in you, it's best to acknowledge it, so you can recognize the signs in good time. You might even see it coming before your gut does and so avoid an attack of IBS. So take a deep breath, and (unless you are reading someone else's copy of the book) check off all those things that pertain to you. Only when you can face up to them and recognize them will you be able and willing to take steps to change things.

After reading the rest of the book and learning a few new techniques for handling stress, you may come back to this list a few weeks later and find that you have managed to avoid some destructive patterns and behaviors. For example, if you drive more impatiently when things pile up on you, and if you can recognize this, then next time you're about to shout at another motorist or blow your horn, you could catch yourself and say, "Hold on a minute, I'm obviously feeling stressed out, so I'd better do something about it—soon." With any luck, in a month's time you'll look back on four weeks of peaceful driving (and maybe a peaceful digestive system), and know that it works to bring your behavior and emotions under control.

## Stress and Your Irritable Bowel

> IBS patients are given diagnoses that appear to be vague, therapy that appears to be ineffective, and a prognosis that seems to be uncertain; meanwhile they are left with symptoms that suggest the possibility of undetected gastrointestinal disease.
>
> —From *Digestion 45*, 1990

The symptoms of IBS can be worrying (abdominal pain, erratic bowel habits, a bloated and distended abdomen, mucus with stools or by itself), and it isn't surprising that many people do worry that they have some serious disease like colitis or even cancer. Having started to worry, their anxiety can make the bowel behave even more irritably, and a vicious circle is set up.

If you are worried about the assorted collection of symptoms that make up this syndrome, it would be a good idea to go to your doctor and get it properly diagnosed; if you don't, the anxiety itself could be making it worse. Rest assured that IBS is not life threatening, and there is no known connection between it and any serious bowel disease. It may be painful, embarrassing, disruptive to your daily life, and a real nuisance, but it won't kill you.

For many people, though, what *will* make IBS worse is stress. This could be any of the stresses of everyday living or the stress of IBS itself. As you will know, having IBS can impose a whole range of extra stresses, particularly when you are away from home:

—Will there be a toilet where I'm going?

—How will I manage if there isn't one?

—What will other people think if I have to go to the toilet several times?

—Will the meal contain any of the things that disagree with me?

—Will my stomach rumbling or breaking wind cause embarrassment?

It's quite possible to start worrying about any one of these things the moment you know you are going on vacation, staying with friends, having a business lunch, or meeting someone in a strange place. You worry that you'll feel tense, and then you start feeling tense. At that point the muscles in your large bowel start to contract extra vigorously, you get abdominal pain and possibly diarrhea, and your original anxiety is reinforced. It becomes all too easy to think, "I can't do this, because if I do I'll get terrible pain and diarrhea," although at this stage the pain and diarrhea are being caused solely by your worry about getting pain and diarrhea. It is an interesting fact that many people start to get the symptoms of IBS before going out for a meal, suggesting that it is the anxiety about eating out rather than the food itself that is the root of the problem.

The quotation from *Digestion* magazine at the beginning of this section continues on to say that feelings of anxiety are ". . . consistent with the state of mind of a patient who is still searching for some rational explanation—and some effective therapy—for his or her symptoms." It then states that this is consistent with the suggestion that these worries are not the cause of IBS but are the result of the IBS being ineffectively managed in the present state of medical knowledge. When the day comes that a cure or effective treatment is found for IBS, it is quite possible that these patients will find their anxiety diminishes, simply because their condition is now understood and treatable.

## Stress and Gut Feelings

All of us notice a connection between fear, emotions, anxiety, and the behavior of our insides, because there are direct nerve pathways between the brain and the intestines. That could explain why there are so many expressions in our language suggesting a link between the emotions and the gut. Consider this imaginary conversation between two women:

*Anna:* How did the promotion interview go?

*Penny:* Oh, fine in the end. I had real butterflies in my stomach all week, but I needn't have worried; I got the job.

*Anna:* That's wonderful news. I had a gut feeling that you would. What's John got to say about all the extra work you'll have to do?

*Penny:* Well, he's not too crazy about it. Even now he keeps bellyaching whenever I have to work late. When I told him I'd been invited to apply for the job, I had an awful feeling in the pit of my stomach that he'd persuade me not to, but he didn't. Anyway, how are things with you? How's your new assistant?

*Anna:* He's doing fine. He's got real fire in his belly and intends to get right to the top. The previous guy just didn't have the stomach for hard work. When I'd finally had a bellyful of him, I managed to get him promoted to the head office!

Even a short snatch of conversation such as this one contains seven phrases linking how we feel to how our insides feel. There are others too: "It gets me right in the gut," "She's got guts," "My stomach turned over," "I can't stomach it," and probably many more. We certainly do connect our insides to our emotions.

A distressed mind can easily lead to an overactive bowel. In research experiments, anger, anxiety, and fear produced greater activity in the guts of IBS patients than it did in other people, possibly because IBS patients may have an unusually direct link between their emotions and the workings of their bowels. It could be caused by the adrenaline that anger and anxiety produces; it could be that the bowel is extrasensitive; but for some reason not yet fully understood, if you have IBS, you are more likely than other people to get digestive problems when you are upset.

## The Vicious Circle—And Breaking It

Once something stressful has happened, your body remembers it, so that the next time that thing happens (or you think it might happen), your body's memory takes over and starts to produce adrenaline in anticipation of that event. Let's imagine that you had an argument with your neighbor. This is something particularly stressful, since you have no choice but to live with your neighbors. During the argument, your level of adrenaline will have risen, and your body will remember this. So next time you see your neighbor (or even think about him or her), adrenaline will come rushing in again, your insides will start to churn, and you start feeling stressed out.

From now on, your aim must be to break this circle. A good starting point is to look at what stresses you out. Try looking at each area of your life in turn. The list that follows presents just a few ideas, but you will want to put in your own ones. Often it is helpful just to acknowledge that something is putting stress on you, especially if up until now you haven't thought about it much or perhaps have even denied it to yourself.

As you look at each item on the list, take time to identify those things that upset you and particularly those that aggravate your IBS. As frankly as you can, write down what it is about you and what it is about others that causes the upset. Then write down one or two steps you could take to improve these things that worry you. If you don't do anything to improve things, they might never improve. Later you can come back to this list and see how you can tackle some of these situations and hopefully start to reduce the number of things that irritate your sensitive bowel.

## WHAT STRESSES ME OUT?
## AT HOME

Arguments with _____

_____

_____

_____

_____

Jobs I have to do _____

_____

_____

_____

_____

Jobs I'd like others to do or share _____

_____

_____

_____

_____

Particular things about my partner or spouse _____

_____

_____

_____

_____

Particular things about my children _____

_____

_____

_____

_____


Particular things about my parents and/or in-laws _____

_____

_____

_____

_____


Particular things about the people I live with _____

_____

_____

_____

_____


Particular things about my neighbors _____

_____

_____

_____

_____


Money worries_____

_____

_____

_____

_____

Concerns about my health, especially _____

_____

_____

_____

_____

Concerns about someone else's health, especially_____

_____

_____

_____

_____

Sexual problems _____

_____

_____

_____

_____

Too much to do _____

_____

_____

_____

_____

Not enough to do_____

_____

_____

_____

_____

Not being valued _____

_____

_____

_____

_____

## AT WORK

Relationships with my boss _____

_____

_____

_____

_____

Relationships with my colleague(s) _____

_____

_____

_____

_____

Relationships with subordinate_____

_____

_____

_____

Relationships with others _____

_____

_____

_____

_____

Lack of money_____

_____

_____

_____

_____

Traveling _____

_____

_____

_____

_____

Job insecurity_____

_____

_____

_____

_____

Sexual harassment _____

_____

_____

_____

_____

Other things _____

_____

_____

_____

_____

## OTHER ASPECTS OF MY LIFE

Leisure activities _____

_____

_____

_____

My body _____

_____

_____

_____

_____

Getting older_____

_____

_____

_____

_____

World events, especially _____

_____

_____

_____

_____

Anything else_____

_____

_____

_____

_____

## THINGS THAT MAKE MY IBS WORSE

Eating out, because _____

_____

_____

_____

_____

Going on vacation, because _____

_____

_____

_____

Meeting new people, because_____

_____

_____

_____

Anticipating some things I have to do, especially _____

_____

_____

_____

_____

Anything else_____

_____

_____

_____

_____

Having identified the things that upset you or make you anxious or angry, write down next to each one why you think this happens. Again, be honest with yourself. No one else will read this, but by facing up to the cause of the problem, you will be better able to manage it.

Next, write down as many ideas as you can think of for improving the situation—things you could do, things you could ask other people to do, ways in which you could seek help, ways in which you could alter your attitude to something—anything, in fact, that might make the situation easier for you to live with.

Only you know how stressful each of these is compared with the others. What is a problem for one person may not be for another. However, you might be interested in a list that was published in 1967 in the *Journal of Psychosomatic Research* of the relative stresses of different events. It is known as the Holmes–Rahe Life Stress Inventory, and this is a very slightly adapted version of it. Check off each of these life events that has happened to you during the last year and add the total:

| LIFE STRESS INVENTORY | |
|---|---|
| Death of spouse | 100 |
| Divorce | 73 |
| Separation | 65 |
| Jail sentence | 63 |
| Death of close family member | 63 |
| Major personal injury or illness | 53 |
| Marriage | 50 |
| Being fired at work | 47 |
| Reconciliation with spouse or partner | 45 |
| Retirement | 45 |
| Major change in the health or behavior of family members | 44 |
| Pregnancy | 40 |
| Sexual difficulties | 39 |

| | |
|---|---:|
| Gaining new family members (through birth, adoption, remarriage, older child moving into the home, and so on) | 39 |
| Major business readjustment (merger, reorganization, bankruptcy, and so on) | 39 |
| Major change in financial state (much worse off or much better off) | 38 |
| Death of a close friend | 37 |
| Changing to a different line of work | 36 |
| Major change in the number of arguments with spouse (more or fewer) | 35 |
| Taking on a large loan (such as mortgage or business loan) | 35 |
| Foreclosure on mortgage or loan | 30 |
| Major change in responsibilities at work (such as promotion, demotion, job transfer) | 29 |
| Son or daughter leaving home | 29 |
| Trouble with in-laws | 28 |
| Outstanding personal achievement | 26 |
| Spouse starts or ends work outside the home | 26 |
| Beginning or ending formal schooling | 26 |
| Major change in living conditions (better or worse) | 25 |
| Trouble with boss | 23 |
| Major change in working hours or conditions | 20 |
| Moving | 20 |
| Moving children to a new school | 20 |
| Major change in type or amount of recreational activities | 20 |
| Taking on a small loan (for a car or TV purchase) | 17 |
| Major change in sleeping habits | 16 |
| Major change in number of family get-togethers (more or less) | 15 |
| Major change in eating habits (more or less food, change in diet, change in times of eating) | 15 |
| Going on vacation | 13 |
| Christmas | 12 |
| Minor violations of the law (such as traffic offense) | 11 |

A score of 150 or less shows you had relatively little life change, and so have a low susceptibility to stress-induced health breakdown. A score of 150 to 300 implies about a 50 percent chance of a major health breakdown in the next two years. A score above 300 implies an 80 percent chance of a major health breakdown in the next two years, according to the Holmes–Rahe statistical prediction model.

Many of these things are quite outside your control, but if you learn how to cope with stress and how to limit the amount of stress you have in other areas of your life, you have a much better chance of remaining in good health.

## Women and Irritable Bowel Syndrome

If you were to ask the average doctor if Irritable Bowel Syndrome is more common in women or men, he would almost certainly say, "Oh, it's much more common in women." It would probably surprise him to know that he is mistaken. IBS affects men and women in roughly equal numbers, with women outnumbering men only slightly. Yet most of the patients he sees with IBS are women, and IBS does seem to affect women differently than it does men.

Most women first start to get IBS in their twenties and thirties, whereas men typically start earlier. Women have headaches, backaches, and the typical IBS symptoms listed in Chapter 1. Whereas men are more likely to get diarrhea, women more commonly have constipation. This can be particularly troublesome, as women often find an overly full rectum more painful than men do.

Many women notice changes in their bowel habits during the menstrual cycle. This is probably due to hormonal changes and can result in either diarrhea or constipation. In addition, women often find their irritable bowel is worse during menstruation and during sexual intercourse.

Women with undiagnosed IBS are often referred to a gynecological clinic, where their pain will be discussed but their bowel habits are probably not. This simply delays the correct diagnosis and often leads to unwarranted surgery. Of course, since the pain is due to an irritable bowel rather a gynecological cause, the problem is usually just as bad after the operation as it was before. (Men with IBS pain will probably face removal of the appendix, which is equally unlikely to cure the problem.)

The working woman, whatever her job, has particular stresses. Women often have more monotonous jobs than men, and boredom—whether from work or from being "just a housewife"—is stressful. If she is a high-powered executive, she may feel guilty and selfish asserting her wishes, in contrast with men in the same position who tend to thrive on exerting power and control. She may feel she has to work harder and more effectively than her male colleagues just to hang on to her job. If, in addition to this, a woman has a husband and children, she may feel additional guilt at neglecting her traditional role as homemaker; or she may feel stress when she doesn't neglect it and tries to fulfill several roles at once.

Most books on stress are written with men in mind, usually highly stressed out businessmen. And so the solutions are geared more to men than to women. Yet women have just as much stress as men (albeit of a different kind) and just as many stress-related diseases, but neither the women themselves nor their doctors seem to take them as seriously. Whereas a man might have lots of tests and is then told to have a complete rest, women are more likely to be prescribed tranquilizers and told, "Don't worry, relax, it's nothing a good night's sleep won't cure."

Often women have come across the condescending attitude of some (particularly older) male doctors—"Don't be silly, dear lady." "We have got a vivid imagination, haven't we?" "You really do ask too many questions, my dear." If you have a doctor who is feeding you lines like these, you might be more at ease with a younger doctor or with a female doctor. Doctors are not God—they are just ordinary, fallible people like you and me. You have every right to regard them as your equals, to ask them questions and expect courteous answers, and to receive from them as much respect as you give them.

Stress among women is also caused by being too anxious to please others, being afraid to displease others, or unnecessarily tolerating unfair or unpleasant situations.

For example, a working husband may spend his lunch hour having a leisurely meal, drive home in the car at the end of the day, put his feet up for a while when he gets home, and then spend the evening watching television or doing whatever he wants to do. Children, if he has them, may make very little difference to this routine.

In contrast, his working wife spends her lunch hour shopping and waiting in line, gets the supper started right away, and probably wades through a pile of laundry before bedtime. If she has children, she may have to accept a less interesting job because it fits in with school hours, and it is she who is expected to take time off work if the children are ill. It is also the grown-up daughter who generally looks after elderly parents.

And let us think a minute about family vacations. Does the husband spend his holiday answering the phone, working on a production line, attending business meetings, and all the things he does during a normal working day? Certainly not! Yet each year millions of wives take self-catering "vacations," during which they do exactly what they do at home—shop, cook, clean, often in more difficult surroundings. At the end of the vacation, I wonder who returns the more rested!

At work women are more likely to have to cope with low pay and the sometimes sexist, condescending attitudes of male colleagues—"Don't you worry your pretty little head about that."

Not content with this, we women really are experts at self-reproach. Given half a chance, we will feel guilty—either because we like or don't like our work, or because we aren't on top of things in our personal life. For those of us who are working mothers, we feel guilty because we are not home being a "homemaker," don't give husband and children as much time as we "should," and perhaps honestly speaking, sometimes would rather be at work than at home. Those of us who do stay home worry that we don't contribute financially and that our days are filled doing trivial things. We are wonderful at feeling guilty if we dare to relax, don't do something we ought to have done, or fall short of the ideals we set for ourselves.

So what can you—a young woman, an older woman, a woman with or without husband and children—do about all this? After all, the more you can make some positive changes, the more likely you are to keep your irritable bowel under control.

—Write down on paper all the things that cause you stress. Then decide which ones can be changed by some action on your part and which you must accept and learn to live with. The more you can get rid of, the more inner resources you will have left to cope with the rest.

—From today onwards accept that it's OK to relax, to make some space for yourself. Give yourself permission to take time off, to fall short of your ideals, and to make changes at work or at home that will allow this. Decide from today onwards that it's quite all right to be a working mother, an assertive career woman, a stay-at-home wife, or whatever role you see yourself in.

—Be good to yourself. You are entitled to as much rest, recreation, and personal space as everyone else. Using your most nonaggressive manner, let other people realize this.

—If you have children, encourage them to cook, iron their clothes, do the washing up, put the family's clothes away, and so on. Enjoy the fact that they are doing it, thank them, and don't worry that it might not be done as well as you would have done it.

—See if you can persuade your partner to share the domesticity; perhaps he can share the ironing, shopping, and cooking? Is he no good at cooking? Well perhaps you weren't that good at it when you got together, and you just had to learn. Couldn't he learn, too?

—Try to establish a routine where everyone shares the domestic duties. Or have you, perhaps, built up your own little empire where no one else feels able, capable, or welcome to do these things, and then do you wonder why you are left to do it all while they watch television, play football, or go out?

—At work, is it you who gets saddled with the coffee-making, washing up, running errands, and so on, just because you are a woman? If you have a job that is of similar importance to a man's, try to get the men to do some of these jobs. Instead of the men saying, "Jane, sweetie, just go out and get me some cigarettes, will ya, hon?" see if you can get them to say, "Jane, I'm going out for some cigarettes, can I get you anything?"

—If your IBS gets worse around the time of your periods, be sure to do relaxation exercises then.

—When you do take time off, enjoy it. There's no need to offer excuses to everyone, simply a quiet explanation. Don't spoil this time by feeling guilty about it. Nor should you expect those around you to feel annoyed with you— they almost certainly won't, unless you become so guilty and defensive it provokes them into annoyance.

—Indulge yourself sometimes, without feeling that such self-indulgence is bad.

—When you find yourself thinking, "I really should," say, "It's all right not to."

—Learn first aid and basic home health management, so you don't worry or panic about illness and accidents. Learn how to replace a fuse, change a plug, change a tire, put up a shelf, turn off the electricity and water main, and similar things so you are not dependent on other people who may not be there when you need them. Make sure you understand the family finances, so you don't fear being left alone to cope.

## Irritable Bowel Syndrome and Your Family

Is Irritable Bowel Syndrome hereditary? Probably not. Can it run in families? Yes.

This may seem contradictory. *Hereditary* means it is inherited genetically from your ancestors, and there is very little you can do to prevent yourself from getting it. Current evidence suggests heredity plays only a minor part in IBS. For example, it is much more common in firstborns that in others, and if it were strongly hereditary, it would occur more evenly among all children of a family.

There are, however, several reasons why IBS might run in families. Firstly, members of the same family may have the same type of personality, and this personality may increase their vulnerability to stress. Secondly, members of the same family may have the same sort of diet, and this may increase the chance that they will all be, say, constipated. Thirdly, members of the same family may treat that constipation in the same way: wrongly.

Let us suppose that your elderly great-aunts were permanently constipated. (Though I don't suppose this was ever something they talked about!) This might have been because they got very little exercise, ate a bland diet with no dietary fiber, and took regular doses of liquid paraffin or other purgatives every day "for regularity." So this constipation was not something that they had inherited or passed on to you. It was directly linked to their way of life.

If your father had IBS, could this be because he was often under a lot of stress, never relaxed, and ate very little dietary fiber? Would he pick it up after a bout of "holiday tummy"?

So rather than heredity, a shared physical and emotional environment is more likely to account for the fact that some of your close relatives may have IBS. That said, there are two factors that may run in families. One is intolerance to dairy products caused by an enzyme deficiency, and the other is an abnormality of the smooth muscle of the colon. Both of these may be present with IBS, and both may be hereditary.

"Indigestion" problems often start in infancy. The colicky baby may become a constipated child, frequently complaining of stomach aches. As a young teenager, he or she may have irregular bowel habits, still with occasional stomach aches. By the time the child reaches late teens or early twenties, he or she may even have had an operation to try to get to the bottom of the problem. But if the problem is IBS, removing the appendix is certainly no solution!

Some children who get IBS may develop initial symptoms after a stressful event such as a bout with the flu or problems at school or at home. Though stress itself doesn't cause IBS, it can trigger symptoms. A survey in London, England, found that children with recurring abdominal pain often came from families in which members had a similar problem. In addition, members of their families had more operations than usual and visited the doctor more often. The families studied tended to have more marital breakdowns and other forms of stress than other families. Think carefully about whether your family life contributed to stomach problems in you and, in turn, whether your family life may be giving your children stomach problems, because about one-third of adults with IBS have had the symptoms since childhood.

Among children, IBS tends to show itself in one of two ways—with diarrhea or pain. When diarrhea predominates as a symptom (which is more common with children under the age of three), the condition is marked by alternating diarrhea and constipation, with little pain. In children over age five, pain is a more common symptom than diarrhea. A crampy pain around the navel or in the lower left region of the abdomen gets worse with eating and better after the child passes a stool or gas. In addition to these symptoms, children may also complain of headaches, nausea, or mucus in the stool. If a child stops eating in hopes of avoiding pain, weight loss, dizziness and other related problems may occur. Treatment for children usually emphasizes dietary changes, increasing fiber and decreasing fat, as well as training the child to empty the bowels regularly at specific times of the day.

Quite a lot of research has been done into how people with IBS were treated as children, to see if past history offers any clues to present problems. Probably the most interesting finding is that, as children, they were more likely to be allowed to stay home from school if they had stomach aches than if they had other disorders such as headaches. Also, if they had stomach aches they were often given gifts or special food, but not when they had other complaints. It is easy to see how a child can quickly associate stomach aches with parental sympathy, gifts, and days off school.

Of course, none of this may apply to you. Your IBS may have appeared for the first time in adulthood. But if you have IBS, then there is a chance that it may be in part due to the way you were brought up. It's also possible that your son or daughter may get it because of the sort of physical and emotional household that he or she is being or has been brought up in. It's worthwhile looking at the way you bring up your children, to see if you are forming habits now that may give them IBS later.

Here's an exercise you can do. Spend a few minutes writing down on a piece of paper every word that describes you, both good and bad. The list might include such uncomplimentary descriptions as *stupid, selfish, uncoordinated, not academic, fat,* or *gawky.* Then put a check mark against any word that was used by your parents or teachers to describe you. You may be surprised to see how many unhelpful descriptions of yourself you are carrying around from your childhood.

Are you doing the same thing to your children? Are you perhaps unwittingly turning them into vulnerable or aggressive people by the way you treat them? Are you lowering their self-esteem and thereby reducing their ability to cope with life, making them more prone to stress and more likely to get a stress-related condition such as IBS?

Would you recognize stress in your child? Early warning signs are the same ones you see in adults: fatigue, difficulty with concentration, irritability, and so on. Of course, any of these can be just part of the normal process of adolescence and nothing in particular to worry about. But most parents have a built-in sense of knowing when something is wrong, so listen to your inner voice and try to help your children if you think they are particularly stressed out.

If your child has persistent stomach aches, get it properly diagnosed by a doctor. After all, the outlook is better if it is caught early. If the diagnosis is IBS, you can help your child (or children) greatly in the following ways:

—Allow them time and space to visit the toilet in peace and without embarrassing comments about noise, smell, and the time they take.

—Because children and young people are so easily put off using the toilet, make yours as attractive as possible—carpet, curtains, interesting things on the wall, a shelf of books and magazines, or a radio or cassette player.

—Be aware if they are feeling anxious about anything and take it seriously without turning it into a momentous world issue.

—Teach them simple methods of relaxation.

—Make sure they eat healthy meals, with plenty of dietary fiber, and without feeling rushed. Encourage them to eat at reasonable times and in a reasonable way.

—Establish a good routine at the start of the day, allowing time for a wholesome, leisurely breakfast and time to establish regular bowel habits.

—Help them to feel comfortable discussing bowel habits with you. Don't provoke their embarrassment; keep the subject low-key so that they don't become obsessive about it.

—If they complain of persistent stomach aches, get them checked by the doctor, but don't reward them or make stomach aches a constant subject of discussion.

These are ways directly related to IBS in which you can help. But there are other ways, too. The ideas that follow are from various sources, including several pieces of research on IBS personality, and I list them without any sense of being holier-than-thou. Bringing up children is difficult, but you may believe, as I do, that helping to build the generation that follows us is one of the most important (and undervalued) jobs in the world. If you can follow most of these ideas, you will have children you can find joy in—and they probably won't develop IBS!

—Remember that many people with IBS have had a series of events in their lives that caused stress and led them to feel anxious and hopeless. Do all you can to make sure this does not happen to your children.

—Show love openly to your adolescent children. This will help them grow into loving adults.

—Really listen to what your children say. Then say something encouraging, not something instructive, competitive, or belittling.

—Many children believe they are loved only if they are winners. So praise your children for the effort they make, not just for their achievement. Make them feel proud of whatever they achieve, however small it seems to you.

—Help them find their own solutions to problems. Don't force your views on them. When talking with them, see how seldom you can use the word "I."

—Cut down on the verbal advice. Instead, display by your own example the sort of person you would like your son or daughter to become. Most children model themselves on their parents for much of their childhood.

—Some hard-driving parents never let their children win at family games because they believe this instills the right competitive attitude for life. But it can produce a child who grows into an angry adult, always driving for achievement. Introduce your child to sports without leagues and trophies to be constantly striving for.

—When you play games with your children, end each session at a point of confidence and success; don't continue to exhaustion or failure.

—Many parents cannot stand being corrected, criticized, or challenged by their children. Practice saying to your children, "Yes, you're right about that, and I'm wrong."

—Encourage them to express their emotions. Even boys can cry.

—Allow children to make mistakes; in recovering from these mistakes they gain self-confidence.

—Never hit your children. If you hit them a lot, you will quite probably turn them into aggressive adults, with your sons growing into violent men who hit their wives and children, and your daughters growing into depressive women who find it difficult to show love to their children. This is how the cycle continues.

—Be aware of how your children see themselves in relation to others. What are they proud or ashamed of? In what ways would they like to be different? If children feel they are failing to live up to your expectations, they may become stressed out. If necessary, revise your expectations to fit in with how things really are.

—Encourage your children to feel comfortable with themselves as they are. Adolescents are easily deflated by criticism, by body image, by physical imperfections. Depending on how these feelings are handled, they could become shy and withdrawn or aggressive and hostile. Downplay the significance of acne, weight, and so on. Try to be aware of the long-term effects your comments and off-the-cuff statements can have on your children's perceptions of themselves.

Keep in mind these quotations:

—From Goethe: "We can't form our children on our own concepts; we must take them and love them as God gives them to us."

—From Kahil Gibran: "You may give them your love but not your thoughts, for they have their own thoughts. You may house their bodies but not their souls, for their souls dwell in the house of tomorrow, which you cannot visit, not even in your dreams. You may strive to be like them, but seek not to make them like you, for life goes not backward nor tarries with yesterday."

# 4

## *Antidotes to IBS*

# Reducing Your Resistance to Stress

Reducing your resistance to stress is not at all the same thing as giving in to it. When you give in, your physical and mental health take a turn for the worse; when you reduce your resistance to it, you should notice an improvement in your health in general and your IBS in particular.

In the previous chapter, you wrote down those things that stress you out, the reasons you think this happens, and some possible ways you might start to improve things. Look again at that list and imagine one situation that upset you. Let's suppose it was an argument with your neighbor: As you remember it, your muscles will start to tense up, your breath will become quicker and more shallow, and your insides will churn. Now take a deep breath in and out, unclench your hands, lower your shoulders, relax your jaw, and breathe quietly and evenly. Imagine yourself seeing your neighbor next time and being quite calm. You are talking to him, but even if he is angry with you, your hands and shoulders are relaxed and your breath is coming quietly and deeply. You are talking in a quiet, calm voice. His anger is not getting to you. Continue to imagine yourself in control of this situation, feeling untroubled and inwardly quiet.

Try this with all the things on your list, starting with the ones that bother you least. See yourself feeling calm and quiet in situations that had bothered you only slightly. When you feel confident that the method works, move on to more difficult situations. Allow yourself plenty of time for each, maybe tackling one each day or two. The important thing is to override your body's unpleasant memory of that situation. Some things may never completely resolve themselves, but if they can trouble you less than they did before, you will feel better emotionally and physically.

One way to reduce unnecessary anger and anxiety is to cut down any negative "self-talk." Most of us talk to ourselves from time to time, some people more than others. What are you saying to yourself? And what effect is it having on you and the tranquillity of your bowel? Are you reinforcing your anger, for example, by going over and over in your mind the argument with your neighbor and all the things you'd like to say to him now you've had time to think about it? Or are you reinforcing negative images you have of yourself: "I can't do anything right," "Life is so unfair to me," "It must be my fault," "I know that situation is going to make me anxious," and so on.

You can replace these self-destructive thoughts with more positive ones that reduce your anger and anxiety and make you feel better in yourself. The first step is to stop each thought dead in its tracks. As soon as you start to recall that argument or anything else that arouses an unpleasant feeling in you, stop! Just like that. End of thought. Consciously make your mind a complete blank for a few moments, and then fill it with a pleasant positive thought. Force yourself to do it. If you can't immediately think of a pleasant thought, recite a poem or a nursery rhyme or sing a song—anything to cancel out those negative thoughts.

It is all too easy to dig a little groove in your mind that instinctively grinds away with negative thoughts. And the deeper the groove, the harder it is to get out of it. So you have to recognize the thought the moment it happens and force yourself into thinking something pleasant and helpful. Before long, you'll be surprised how seldom you think those useless thoughts; that groove will have disappeared, and you will be on the way to reducing the level at which things upset you.

## Measure Your Resistance

You can measure your ability to cope with stress by completing the test below, which was developed by Lyle H. Miller and Alma Dell Smith of Boston University Medical Center. The test measures the degree to which your way of life supports you and bolsters resistance to stress. Rate yourself for each of the 20 items on the scale from 1 (almost always) to 5 (never) according to how often they apply.

| How often are the following statements true for you? | Almost Always | Most Times | Someimes | Rarely | Never |
|---|---|---|---|---|---|
| 1. My health is good (including eyesight, teeth, and so on) | 1 | 2 | 3 | 4 | 5 |
| 2. My income meets my basic expenses. | 1 | 2 | 3 | 4 | 5 |
| 3. I am about the right weight or my build and height. | 1 | 2 | 3 | 4 | 5 |
| 4. I give and receive affection regularly. | 1 | 2 | 3 | 4 | 5 |
| 5. I express my feelings when angry or worried. | 1 | 2 | 3 | 4 | 5 |
| 6. I have fewer than three caffeinated drinks (coffee, tea, cocoa, or cola) a day. | 1 | 2 | 3 | 4 | 5 |
| 7. I take part in regular social activities. | 1 | 2 | 3 | 4 | 5 |

| | Almost Always | Most Times | Sometimes | Rarely | Never |
|---|---|---|---|---|---|
| 8. I eat at least one full, well-balanced meal a day. | 1 | 2 | 3 | 4 | 5 |
| 9. I do something just for pleasure at least once a week. | 1 | 2 | 3 | 4 | 5 |
| 10. There is at least one relative within 50 miles of home on whom I can rely. | 1 | 2 | 3 | 4 | 5 |
| 11. I have some time alone during the day. | 1 | 2 | 3 | 4 | 5 |
| 12. I get seven or eight hours of sleep at least four nights a week. | 1 | 2 | 3 | 4 | 5 |
| 13. My religious beliefs give me strength. | 1 | 2 | 3 | 4 | 5 |
| 14. I exercise hard enough to work up a sweat at least twice a week. | 1 | 2 | 3 | 4 | 5 |
| 15. I have a network of friends and acquaintances. | 1 | 2 | 3 | 4 | 5 |
| 16. I discuss problems such as house-work and money with other members of the household. | 1 | 2 | 3 | 4 | 5 |
| 17. I have at least one friend I can talk to about personal affairs. | 1 | 2 | 3 | 4 | 5 |
| 18. I smoke no more than 10 cigarettes a day. | 1 | 2 | 3 | 4 | 5 |
| 19. I organize my time well. | 1 | 2 | 3 | 4 | 5 |
| 20. I have fewer than five alcoholic drinks a week. | 1 | 2 | 3 | 4 | 5 |

Add up your total score. A score of 45 or less shows high resistance to stress and a healthy way of life. A score between 45 to 55 indicates that you may be susceptible to the effects of stress and could benefit from adjusting certain aspects of your daily life. If the score is over 55, stress could be a serious risk, calling for a reappraisal of your general way of life.

It's unlikely that you will be able to correct every single problem on the list, so begin by working on those things you can control. For example, you may not be able to do much about the fact that you have no relatives within 50 miles or that you have no religious beliefs. But you could compensate by working on as many as possible of the other ones, even if you hadn't thought about them before. Perhaps you could make time alone for yourself each day or do something just for pleasure at least once a week.

## Other Things You Can Do about Stress

This section is full of ideas for reducing stress and for coping with the stress that you can't get rid of. Some of the ideas may not appeal to you or be of any help; others may seem particularly helpful. Even if you cannot remove all the causes, you can at least reduce the more harmful effects.

There are five important steps you can take to better manage your stress:

1. Recognize the signs that show you are under stress.

2. Be aware of what causes stress in your life.

3. Identify what you find relaxing and develop some techniques for winding down.

4. Try, if possible, to remove or at least reduce the number of stressful things in your life.

5. Anticipate and prepare yourself for those things you just have to put up with.

First of all, learn to recognize signs of stress in yourself. In all of us, stress shows in one way or another. How does it show itself in you? Do you, for example, sit on the edge of your chair, tap your fingers on the table or on the steering wheel, bang your knees together, or clench your hands or teeth? Do you get a headache, shoulder pains, a sense of restlessness, or fatigue? Think about how you express stress, so you can recognize it the moment it appears.

Next, recognize what causes these stress signals. What makes you tense? Your IBS probably comes and goes in response to particular events. Can you recognize in advance that a particular event will trigger it? Or if it doesn't recur until after a stressful event, could you have anticipated the stress and done something to prevent it?

Take time to consider what causes IBS to recur for you. Perhaps you can now say, "Yes, it always gets worse when . . . ." If you can do that, you are making progress.

A small amount of stress can be beneficial, but too much can be harmful. In your case, stress above a particular level or of a particular type triggers your irritable bowel. Only you can tell where those thresholds are, but you must now work to keep the stress below the level that triggers IBS for you. How can you do that?

Go back to the list you compiled in Chapter 3 where you jotted down which situations give you the most trouble, which ones you get most anxious or agitated about. Now write down why you think this happens. Does your bowel get irritable in anticipation of these situations, or afterward? What other physical symptoms do you notice? Write it all down. Your body will remember a stressful situation, so the next time that situation occurs, your body will start to produce adrenaline in anticipation of it. (It's like our prehistoric friend, *Homo sapiens*, on his regular meetings with the four-toed mammoth.)

Now sit down, look again at that list, and imagine each situation in turn. As you imagine it, see yourself being relaxed in that situation; lower your shoulders, unclench your hands and your jaw, and breathe deeply and evenly until you can think about that situation without anxiety. Do this several times.

It is obvious that you are going to have to make changes. After all, if you go on as you are, your IBS will always be there, ready to pounce when things get difficult. Yet it's never too late to make changes of any sort. Start today. Say to yourself, "From this moment on I am going to be different in such-and-such a way." Then stick to it. Nothing dramatic, nothing that you can't keep up; start in a small way, one step at a time. Making these kinds of changes is an ongoing process and if you fail, you should just try again.

What follows is a list of ideas, set down at random, any of which may be just right for you. For many of them you will probably say, "Well, that's easier said than done; there's no way I can do that." Only you know whether this is really true, or whether, with a little effort and planning, you could do it if it meant relief from your irritable bowel.

—As you sit at a desk, factory bench, kitchen table, or in the car, bus, or train, get into the habit of noticing muscle tension in your feet, thighs, abdomen, shoulders, hands, neck, mouth, and forehead. Then relax. Although you will put aside extra time to relax in peace and quiet, it is important you are also able to relax at any time of day, in any situation—in a bus line, traffic jam, office, restaurant, wherever you are.

—Avoid prolonged driving (which can raise your blood pressure and get you terribly wound up inside).

—Avoid tight deadlines. It is better to work a longer day without tension than a shorter day with it.

—Have modest goals, both professional and personal. Do you really need all that overtime money? Are the things you buy with your money really essential to your inner happiness? Keeping up with the Joneses is not a healthy habit. Overambition can cause great stress to you and your family.

—Learn to like people for who they are rather than for what they have. Have as friends people who like you for who you are, not for what you have. After all, you may not always have whatever it is they like.

—Bear in mind that more stress is caused by things left undone than by things done. Be sure to do the things that really matter, so you aren't worrying because you haven't done them.

—Reduce major tasks to manageable ones. Plan your time effectively. Divide each day's tasks into priority categories A, B, and C. Do the ones marked A, and only if you have time do B and C. If not, leave them. They could be tomorrow's priority A tasks. There will always be some things that don't get done, so aim to make sure that these are the least important tasks.

—Learn to delegate. Ask your subordinates at work to do something you were going to do and then let them get on with it. Ask your children to do some household jobs, and don't keep checking up on them. Even if the job is not done perfectly or quickly, does it really matter all that much? A job is hardly ever ruined by being done too slowly.

—Giving and receiving love is a sign of strength, not of weakness. Show physical affection to family and close friends. A hug or a touch on the arm is a wonderful way of showing you care for someone. Have confidence that you can touch people without communicating any sexual overtones. Other people do it all the time, so no one will think it odd if you do it, too.

—Develop a hobby that is relaxing and noncompetitive. Give time to it.

—Get regular exercise. It lifts the spirits, works off the cares that pile up on you, revives your outlook on life, gives you more energy, and makes it easier to cope with stress. But keep it noncompetitive if you can. Racquetball may keep you fit, but it won't help your irritable bowel one little bit if you are determined to beat everyone you play against. The best forms of noncompetitive exercise are swimming, running, outdoor cycling, and brisk walking.

—Pause several times a day to do nothing, to think of pleasant things, to meditate. Promise a few minutes a day to yourself. It will do wonders for your gut.

—Stroking the cat is very soothing. Heart specialists often recommend it as a way of reducing blood pressure!

—Try not to have disruptions in too many areas of your life at once. If you are having problems at work, don't stir things up at home. If you have problems at home, try to make sure all is well at work and with your friends. If your leisure-time activities are getting you all bothered, keep things calm at home and work.

—Every time something really irritates you or arouses feelings of anger or hostility, write it down at the time. Do this every day, and then at the end of the week read what you have been writing down in the preceding days. Do you feel that you have been getting irrationally angry over remarkably trivial things? Do all those things that got you so cross at the time still seem so important several days later?

—We all have a limited ability to withstand stress, and people with IBS possibly have a more limited ability than others. So don't waste the reserves you do have on pointless anger and hostility. If you do, there will be nothing left when you need it. And recognize that anger is not only there when you show it by losing your temper. You may be the sort of person who keeps things inside you; that doesn't mean you don't feel angry, only that you don't show it outwardly.

—Anger harms you more than it harms the person whom you are angry with. There's an old Chinese proverb (there always is!) that says, "Before you seek revenge on your enemy, you must first dig two graves."

—Choose your own goals. Don't necessarily accept the goals set for you by your parents, your partner, your teacher, your employer. If you fail to live up to goals set by other people, this can cause great anxiety.

—Really listen to what other people say. Listen without criticism, without trying to improve on it, without using the word "I" in your reply. Talking increases blood pressure ever so slightly, and listening decreases it, so spend more time listening than talking, and you will feel calmer.

—Try not to bottle up your emotions. If people take advantage of you, you may find that attending a self-assertiveness course will teach you to express what you feel in a calm, nonthreatening way. This will benefit every aspect of your life. Your local library or adult education center may have details.

—Most of us like people who make us feel good and increase our self-esteem and dislike those who make us feel small, incompetent, or foolish. What effect do you have on family, friends, workmates, those around you? Think about this very carefully.

—Is your home "designed for the way you live today"? In other words, is it set up for a hurried lifestyle? Instant food, microwave oven, a breakfast bar where you perch as you gobble your food, a fast car that encourages you to rush everywhere, clocks in every room, lots of time-saving gadgets . . . what does this say about the way you live? Slow down. Relax.

—Maintain a balance of work and family time and responsibilities. Try not to let one area of your life dominate all the others.

—Share the decision-making; don't take all life's burdens on your shoulders. You'll be amazed how well other people can cope if you trust them to. If someone makes a mistake, always give him or her another chance.

—Give your opinions in an honest, loving, and nonthreatening way.

—If you have problems and anxieties, talk about them. Don't bottle them up. Share your feelings with a friend, and likewise take time to listen to your friend's worries.

—When you know an event is coming that you will find stressful and that may well trigger your irritable bowel, take extra time for breathing exercises and meditation. Visualize in your mind the stressful event and see yourself in control and feeling calm about it; work at it until you no longer feel that knot in your stomach.

—Forgive, even if you find it difficult to forget; don't hold grudges. Try to see situations from other people's viewpoints and understand why they behave as they do. If you had been in the other person's shoes, might you have done the same thing?

—Stress doesn't just result from pressure outside—it also results from your perception of something as stressful. If you have conditioned yourself to regard trivial situations as threatening, then every time those situations happen, stress is triggered in you. So rethink what gets you all worked up. Is it really a life-and-death issue if dinner is served late? If a driver overtakes you on the freeway? Do those around you perhaps feel you are making a mountain out of a molehill? They may be right.

—People like people who help people, so see how much you can help others. People also like people whom they help, so receive help willingly and graciously. By making others feel good about themselves, they will feel good toward you.

—Share your feelings, ideas, and frustrations with someone you can trust. If there is no one in your life whom you can trust, why is that? What does it tell you about yourself?

—Have you noticed that the things we complain about in other people are usually the things we ourselves are guilty of?

—When you are wrong, apologize. Don't be the sort of person of whom others say, "She just never could admit she was wrong." If you are not used to it, it is extraordinarily difficult, but it becomes easier with practice and has a wonderful effect on relationships. Start with small mistakes—"I'm sorry I spilled the tea"—and build up to the larger issues: "I'm sorry I wasn't there when you wanted me to be"; "I'm sorry I didn't give you more of my time"; or even simply "I'm sorry—I was wrong."

—Whatever your position in life, consider taking a course in stress management. You will probably learn one or more of the following techniques: using various forms of relaxation to reduce or control the level at which you start to feel angry or anxious; recognizing and preventing what triggers tension in you; changing your perceptions of different situations, so you no longer see them as threatening; not feeling helpless about your condition.

—At the end of each day, spend time doing relaxation exercises. And recall each episode of the day in which you felt things get on top of you, or you did not react as well as would have liked to. Ask yourself, "How could I have handled that better?" Ask yourself whether you have eaten inappropriately or done other things to make you feel rushed or stressed. Was it necessary? How could you have avoided it? Resolve to make whatever changes will prevent the same thing from happening again.

> —Make a list of those things that help you to wind down and relax. Here are some ideas to get you started, but you will be able to add many more of your own.

| Relaxing Activity | How Often I Do It | How Often I'd Like to Do It |
|---|---|---|
| Watching TV | | |
| Soaking in a bath | | |
| Listening to music | | |
| Reading | | |
| Going for a walk | | |
| Talking to a friend | | |
| Fishing | | |
| Swimming | | |
| Playing a sport | | |
| Gardening | | |
| Going to a café or bar | | |
| Lying in the sun | | |
| Playing with the children | | |
| Getting out of the house | | |
| Jogging | | |
| Sleeping | | |
| Having my hair done | | |
| Playing an instrument | | |
| Writing letters | | |
| Cooking | | |
| Painting | | |
| Walking the dog | | |

Next to each item write down how often you do it and then how often you would like to do it. If there is a significant difference between these two factors, write down why that might be and what you might be able to do about it. What arrangements could be made? Who could help you? When could you start doing this?

For your general health and for your IBS, you should put time aside regularly to do the things that relax you. This isn't something that should be dismissed as not all that important, something that you will get around to one day. If you are not getting enough opportunities to do these pleasurable things, start thinking what you can do today to make some changes.

## Planning for Change

How do you feel about change? Does it excite you? Do you dread it? Do you feel you'd like to change things but are afraid to or don't know how?

You could start by making an action plan. Things don't have to stay as they are. They can change, and you can be the one that makes the changes.

Get out a large sheet of paper and on it draw a picture of your life as you would like it to be in two or three years' time. You could divide it into different areas, such as Home, Work, Leisure, and so on. In each section draw the new you, as you would like to see yourself. Perhaps draw the sort of house you would like to live in, the area you would like to be living in, the kinds of possessions you would like to have (or discard). Draw yourself in the type of job you would like to be doing, where, and with whom. Write down words or phrases or sentences that describe what that area of your life will be like. Include all your deepest ambitions. Try to take at least half an hour on this, longer if possible. Be imaginative and free thinking. Think widely and creatively. Don't be tied down by rational intellectual judgments. Say to yourself, "If I really wanted to, I could be doing anything I wanted":

—Running my own company

—Living in Hawaii

—Reconciled with my sweetheart

—Divorced

—A photographer

—Learning how to hang-glide

—Feeling in control of my IBS

Put down in words or pictures all the things you would like your life to contain, both possible and impossible. Then give yourself permission to want these things.

Now choose one or two that you really would like to be, have, or do in the next twelve months: "In a year from now I'd like to. . . ."

**Filling in the following chart may help you.**

*What do I hope to achieve by this time next year?*

_____

_____

_____

_____

_____

*What obstacles are preventing me from doing this?*

_____

_____

_____

_____

_____

*What am I afraid of?*

_____

_____

_____

_____

_____

*Which of my particular strengths will help me to achieve this?*

_____

_____

_____

_____

_____

*Who could help me? Who could I talk to? Who knows how to do it?*

_____

_____

_____

_____

_____

*What further information do I need to do this?*

_____

_____

_____

_____

_____

*Where is help and advice available?*

_____

_____

_____

_____

_____

*In order to do this, my first step will be*

_____

_____

_____

_____

_____

Having gotten this far, now go ahead and take that first step today if possible. Try to break down those things that are standing in the way of your goal and build up those things that will allow it to happen.

## Your Job

One area of people's lives that seems to cry out for change is their employment. To become employed rather than unemployed; to be self-employed rather than work for someone else, or the other way around; to work shorter or longer hours; to have more or less responsibility, more or less pressure; to work in a different area or environment, or with different people; to do the same thing but differently; or to do something totally, entirely, mind-bendingly different.

More working days are lost each year from stress-related illnesses than from the common cold; in the majority of cases, the job itself is the cause of the stress.

It could be helpful, therefore, for you to carefully consider whether you are in the right job, especially if stress connected with work is making your irritable bowel worse. If your job makes you feel aggressive, hostile, inadequate, or depressed, maybe it's time for a change. If you had a job that suited your personality and temperament, you would probably do it well and be well able to cope. So if you know that you could do your job much better if you really wanted to, but somehow you don't want to, then maybe you are in the wrong job. Most people are reluctant to make a major job change, but if a change is forced upon them (by a layoff, for example), most are amazed at how much happier they are in the new job.

The days are long gone when most people stayed in the same type of job and with the same company for the whole of their working lives. Nowadays, the average person has three quite separate careers, working in at least three jobs in each career. So many people find themselves in the wrong job that three years is the average length of time for staying in any one job.

"But what else can I do?" you ask yourself. "I'm trained to be a water engineer/secretary/dentist/filing clerk/accountant/car mechanic/ machine operator. I don't know any other job. I'm too old (too young) to do something else. I live in the wrong place. I can only work when the children are at school. I need the money this job brings in. I'd love to change, but. . . ."

Whether you are considering moving to a new job or even to a completely new career, a good way to start is to buy or borrow a copy of the career-changer's bible, *What Color Is Your Parachute?* by Richard Nelson Bolles (Ten Speed Press). This book is updated each year and available in most bookstores. There are several manuals on the market that aim to help people find their right niche in life, but this one is probably the most helpful and useful. By taking time to work through it, you will have a good idea of what your strengths and weaknesses are, what matters to you in a job, what is less important, what kind of people you like working with, what sort of job you should be looking for, how to go about getting it, whether retraining would be a good idea, and much, much more. Almost certainly, by the time you have worked conscientiously through the book (which will take days rather than hours), you should have a good idea of what sort of job is right for you.

Other sources of guidance are career counseling centers (look in the *Yellow Pages*), your local adult continuing education career department, or even your local high-school career office. Many local authorities are willing to share their knowledge and information sources with people and some even give access to computer programs that help you to see the direction you might go in. If you are not enjoying your job, think seriously about a change, especially if you think aspects of your job are making your IBS worse.

It is a myth that the high-powered executive suffers the highest levels of stress. Blue-collar workers suffer considerably higher rates of stress than white-collar workers, largely due to the lack of control they have over their work and the lack of interest and purpose they find in it. Stress-related illness is very closely connected with the amount of control and the status you connect with your job, so people whose jobs score badly on these two points are worse off. A job with too few challenges becomes boring, frustrating, and stressful.

A survey in *Which?* magazine in 1977 found that the most satisfied workers tended to be employed by a small firm where they had a responsible position, worked long hours, had lots to do, had some control over what they did, and felt their work was important and mattered to the firm. The survey also included a job satisfaction list, and those jobs that were high on the list were ones in which people had higher-than-average control over how they did the job. With respect to your own job, ask yourself:

—Do I get enough variety in my job?

—Does my job make good use of all my skills?

—Do I get opportunities to make decisions about my work?

—Do I feel valued by those above me?

—Do I feel proud of what I produce?

—Can I take reasonable breaks, such as going to the toilet, when I want to?

If the answer to even one of these questions is no, then your work is probably already a source of stress to you. It might be helpful if you could talk to someone about it, preferably someone who is in a position to make changes or to help you make changes. Maybe your boss has never done the sort of job you do, so she is unaware of its particular stresses.

White-collar workers certainly don't escape lightly either. Many organizations expect their employees to become highly involved in the success of the company and of their job in particular. Heavy investments of time and energy are demanded—working evenings and weekends, traveling away from home on company business, going to work-related social activities, even being willing to move to a different area in the company's interest.

Whatever kind of work you do, there are certain things that can make a job stressful:

—Too much work

—Too little work

—Deadlines

—Unclear goals

—Poor prospects for advancement

—Low pay

—Bureaucracy

—Low status

—Isolation

—Having no clear criteria of success

—Having to make too many decisions

—Not being allowed to make enough decisions

—Physical fatigue

—Excessive travel

—Long hours

—The boss's temperament

—New management style

—Customers, clients, patients who are hostile and demanding

—Feeling trapped

—Relocations

—Layoffs (or fear of them)

—Skills or attitudes that are out of date

—Divided loyalties

—The consequences (monetary and career) of making mistakes

—Boredom

—Shift work

—Mistrust of those in power

—Career plateau

—Workplace politics

—Sexual harassment

—Difficult co-workers

There are also physical factors that cause stress at work:

—An unsuitable desk, chair, stool, workbench

—Work done in an uncomfortable position

—Lighting that is too bright, too dim, or flickering

—Uncomfortable workwear

—Temperature too hot or too cold

—Fumes

—Smoke

—Eye strain

—Noise

If your job includes too many things from these lists, perhaps you should consider a change. Your irritable bowel may be one of the clearest signs you get about how you are feeling about your job. But don't expect any new job to be perfect; almost every job has its downside, and before you leap from the job you know with all its imperfections, it is worth thinking carefully what it is you are trying to get away from. The job may well be extremely stressful, but your personality, beliefs, and attitudes also play an important part in how you manage stress, both at work and at home.

Despite all these potential sources of stress, most people enjoy their jobs most of the time and are happy working at them.

## Meal Times

Here is another area where you could start to do things different-ly. Like so many people, IBS sufferers tend to rush around first thing in the morning, have nothing more nourishing than a cup of coffee for breakfast, then go on to the lunchtime meal of the three Cs: coffee, chips, and a cigarette. Perhaps there is more of the same during the afternoon. Finally, this gastronomically delightful day ends with a large meal of all the wrong things, washed down with rather too much alcohol. Is it any surprise that your bowel protests?

Each new day dawns full of hope that things could be better. Make the most of it and, starting from tomorrow's dawn, decide on some changes.

If your breakfast is always rushed, the only really logical solu-tion (however difficult) is to get up a bit earlier. If you find getting up difficult at any time, you'll probably know that it's not much harder getting up half an hour earlier than getting up at your pre-sent time. What's more, if you had that extra half-hour you could have a much calmer morning for very little extra effort.

So, from tomorrow morning, you will get up thirty minutes earlier than usual! Put aside all thoughts of a mere cup of coffee and a cigarette. Treat yourself to a bowel-friendly breakfast of stewed fruit and muesli with some whole grain toast and one cup of tea or coffee (unless you know that any of these disagree with you). Eat it sitting down on a proper chair at a proper table, not perched on a stool at a breakfast bar, which simply encourages you to finish the meal as quickly as possible and rush on to the next thing. Take your time—after all, you've got thirty extra minutes now.

Your next stop is a visit to the toilet. When you start to eat, a "food-now-entering-stomach" message is sent to the brain, which triggers a whole series of gastrointestinal activities that move each batch of food already in the system on to its next stage. All yesterday's food (and probably the food from the previous day, too) that is in your large intestine gets moving, and inevitably some of it heads for the rectum, producing the familiar "it's-time-to-go" feeling. This feeling is strongest in the morning, after the first meal of the day, and it's an unwise person who ignores these body messages.

When the waste products enter the rectum, they are surrounded by a layer of slippery mucus, which makes the stools easier to pass. If you are so busy in the morning that you won't find time for a visit to the toilet after breakfast, this mucus becomes reabsorbed back into the wall of the rectum, and the stools become hard, dry, and difficult to pass. If you then wait until mid morning or even later, don't be surprised if the simple act of having a bowel movement is not as easy as it should be. So work with your body, not against it.

All the way through the day, listen to what your body is trying to tell you. If you are tired, try to pause for a while to recoup some energy. If you are hungry, eat a nutritious meal and stop when you feel full. Laugh when you are happy; cry when you are sad. Everything we feel is a sign that the body is trying to tell us something. Be aware of it.

If you suspect that the food you eat is contributing in some way to your Irritable Bowel Syndrome, try to make some changes. Once you know which foods make your IBS worse, try hard to avoid them for a while. Give your intestines a rest, and you may find that after a few months you can eat them again without too much difficulty. You are asking for trouble if you continually abuse your insides with food they don't like.

# Daily Stress: The Telephone

How many times a day do you rush to answer the phone, grab the handpiece, and feel your blood pressure rise as you give your name or number? Next time the phone rings, wait. Let it ring two or three times while you spend a moment breathing out with a long outbreath. Let the inbreath come in naturally, then allow yourself another long outbreath. Be aware of any tension in your muscles and consciously relax your face, jaw, neck, shoulders, and hands. Even if you are right beside the phone, pause and prepare yourself to answer it calmly. If you have to make a call that is worrying you, write down in advance the points you wish to make, prepare a list of phrases that you could use, and above all relax and stay calm.

# Daily Stress: The Car

The car is a source of much stress in our lives. Car-related stress comes from two main sources: other drivers (how they drive, how they behave), and pressure of time (traffic jams, red lights, not being able to park, feeling rushed). Here are some ideas for managing the stress these situations can cause:

### OTHER DRIVERS

There's not a lot you as an individual can do to improve how others drive and behave (unless you are a driving instructor, in which case you have marvelous opportunities to teach people to drive calmly and courteously). If you get wound up by other people's driving, try to consider why this is. Why do bus drivers make you feel so angry? Or drivers of a particular make of car? Try to analyze your reactions and see if you can become more accepting.

If you are at the receiving end of a driver's abuse or bad driving, above all *stay calm*. However tempting it might be to retaliate, just relax, accept the situation, and do the simple exercise above. Next time someone shouts at you, tries to show his superiority in some way, or feels the need to prove something at your expense, say to yourself, "This person has a problem. It is his problem. It is not my problem." It is something he must live with, and you mustn't let it bother you. You do not have that problem. Comfort yourself that, if he is a really selfish, aggressive driver, one day he may get his comeuppance!

### PRESSURE OF TIME

This all stems back to allowing enough time for the journey, traffic jams and all. However difficult it may seem, try not to be in a hurry; delays happen on the best-regulated journeys and can cause your blood pressure to increase, your tolerance to decrease, and your intestines to tie themselves in knots. For every journey, allow enough time and then a bit more. Don't say to yourself, "The journey takes twenty minutes. I have to be there at 2:45 p.m., so I'll get ready to leave at 2:25 p.m.," quite forgetting that you must get your things together, get to the car, start the car, drive off, find somewhere to park at the other end, get your things out of the car, and walk into your destination—late!

In an ideal world, your thoughts would go something like this: "I have to be there at 2:45 p.m. It will take about five minutes to get my things together and get to the car; at the other end I must allow five minutes to park, collect my things, and walk to my destination. So I should leave at 2:15 p.m., but in order to be quite relaxed about road work, traffic lights, and a slow truck in front of me, I'll add an extra five minutes and leave at 2:10 p.m." If, in addition, parking is likely to be a problem, add another ten minutes and leave at 2:00 p.m. If you arrive too early, give yourself permission to sit in the car and relax quietly.

## Managing Time

It could be that your IBS is partly caused by the stress of being under pressure of time—trying to fit too many things into too short a time—at home, at work, and even at leisure. Have you thought what changes you could make to give yourself a quieter life?

"Time management" is part of today's jargon—another buzz-word. It involves learning how to make the best use of your time to get everything done without it all getting on top of you. Your library or bookstore may have a book on time-management techniques. A simple approach is to list all the tasks you have to do today, this week, or this month and give them each a priority A, B, or C. If you can't decide whether something should be A or B, put B. If you can't decide whether it should be B or C, put C. Then take all the As and put them in priority: A1, A2, A3, and so on. Do the same for B and C tasks. The priorities can always be changed. Using this technique prevents you spending time on C and then feeling stressed out because you haven't done A. If possible, include some relaxing, pleasant activities into each category. At the end of the period, don't worry if you haven't gotten around to doing the Cs. If they were unimportant, it doesn't matter; if they were important, they will rise to become Bs.

This simple method of time management is effective whether you are the director of a multinational company or a housewife. By using it you are beginning to control your own life rather than letting events control you.

If you often seem to have too much work for the time available, see if you can delegate some of it. Start by making a list of "jobs at work" or "jobs at home" that you would like to hand over to someone else. Think about the time when you could ask this person and the form of words you could use. At home it might be possible to pay someone to do ironing, mow the lawn, clean the car, or decorate the bathroom. Or perhaps you could swap with someone. ("I'll mow your lawn if you'll do my ironing.") If there are any jobs left on your list that you can neither delegate nor swap nor pay someone to do, then perhaps doing them with someone else might make them seem less onerous. You could also do them less often or do them all at once, then "reward" yourself.

In many cases, actually doing the job is not as bad as thinking about it. If you have to do a job you don't like, start with the easy parts of it before going on to the worst part. If you need to stop in the middle, try to choose a point at which it is easy (rather than difficult) to start again. But try to build difficult parts in with the easy parts, because if you do all the easiest parts first you are then left with all the awful parts, which may tempt you to continue putting them off.

Another approach to difficult jobs is to set yourself an exact time (such as 11:30 a.m. on Thursday) and just get on and do it then. Or if it is a tangible job that you don't like (such as ironing), decide you will do it for a certain length of time—say, half an hour—and then stop. Whatever the task, and whatever the method you use to make yourself do it, reward yourself when it is done.

Here are other suggestions for organizing your time more effectively:

—Try to do routine tasks together at the same time once a day, whether it is the ironing at home or routine paperwork at the office. By doing similar tasks in one batch, they will seem to get done quicker.

—When you are doing one job, remove evidence of all the other jobs that are waiting to be done and that are simply a stressful reminder of all the work you still have to do.

—Build into your day some time for important jobs that may crop up unexpectedly, and that simply must be fitted in. If you have no time to fit them in you will soon start to feel stressed out.

—Have a balanced mixture of dull and interesting jobs, of tiring and invigorating ones.

—Make time for yourself each day.

—Try to finish each job before going on to the next; but accept that not all jobs can be finished in the time allowed.

—See if some of the jobs you don't enjoy can be done by someone else who would enjoy doing them.

—When planning your day, plan to do high-energy jobs during the time of day when you are feeling fresh.

—If you are constantly putting off doing something, try to work out why. What exactly don't you like about that job? See if you can get help from some source. But if you really have no option but to do it, then set yourself a fixed time and do it then. The longer you put it off, the longer it hangs over you and becomes a source of stress and worry.

You can probably think of many more ways in which, by doing things differently, you could feel quieter within yourself. Once you have thought about it, have the courage to put these ideas into practice. Just choose one at a time, starting with the easy ones. When you know you can change simple things you will feel motivated to change others.

## Building Personal Resources

In her excellent book *A Woman in Your Own Right—Assertiveness and You*, Anne Dickson identifies four personality types. Although they are all women, the descriptions could fit men just as well:

*Anne* is aggressive. She is loud and forceful and seeks to enhance her own status through belittling others. She doesn't consider other people's views and often alienates those around her. She is determined to win every situation. Anne needs to prove her superiority by putting down other people because underneath she lacks genuine self-esteem. Some people respond aggressively toward her, but most feel defensive; she leaves them feeling hurt, humiliated, and resentful. Many people would like to get back at her but are afraid to for fear of how she will treat them.

*June* is a doormat who tends to opt out of all conflict. She finds it difficult to make decisions, has a persistently negative outlook on life, and sees herself as a victim of unfairness and injustice. She is great at putting herself down. June avoids taking responsibility for making choices in her life and leaves that task for others, which makes them frustrated and resentful.

*Sandra* is indirectly aggressive. She is skilled at hurting and deceiving others without their being able to pinpoint just how she has done it; other people, understandably, feel confused and frustrated. She does not trust herself or anyone else and so will deny her real feelings. She too has low self-esteem, and in order to avoid rejection or hurt she needs to control and manipulate other people when they detect her continuing undercurrent of disapproval. Her main weapon is making others feel guilty in order to get what she wants.

In all three women, their behavior can be traced back to a lack of self-esteem. Perhaps as a child Anne had to prove herself better than other people in order to earn love from her parents and approval from her teachers. She feels no real self-confidence in being herself and so mistrusts others. Maybe June was criticized so often as a child that she is now afraid to show her real feelings. Perhaps Sandra learned that direct straightforward behavior is not encouraged in women and that she must use subtle and devious ways to get what she wants.

Which one, or combination of these, are you? A bit of Anne sometimes? Something of June? Sandra from time to time? Don't feel guilty or blame yourself for whichever you are. Just notice how you tend to behave. Your behavior, like these three women's, almost certainly stems from how you were treated as a child. In which of these categories would you put your mother or your father? How they behaved toward you will have influenced how you see yourself. And it is how you see yourself that determines your behavior toward others.

Anne Dickson's fourth woman is *Selma:*

She is neither aggressive nor passive, but assertive. She respects herself and other people, accepts her own positive and negative qualities, and doesn't feel the need to put others down in order to feel comfortable in herself. She can recognize her needs and ask openly and directly that they be met; if she is refused, she does not feel demolished by the rejection, because her self-esteem is secure.

All these women (and their male equivalents) will obviously feel stress from time to time, but they will handle it quite differently.

The aggressive person (who probably has an underlying insecurity and self-doubt inside that hostile exterior) will tend to express her aggression to those around her. She may do this through outbursts of temper, aggressive driving, or rushing around from A to B—all the time denying that she is stressed out or, even if she acknowledges her stress, telling herself that she hasn't got the time to do anything about it right now. She is possibly coping quite well with her IBS, although she almost certainly denies that it is stress-related.

The passive doormat of a person (whose insecurity and lack of self-esteem is there for all to see) will turn his stress inward into himself, because he is too afraid to risk annoying or hurting other people. He will get tense, work all the harder to prove to himself that he can do it really, inwardly blame other people for his rotten luck, and outwardly put on a brave face so that people might be surprised that he was under any sort of stress. He may feel that people have taken advantage of his good nature and be angry with himself for not having the strength of character to say no.

Both these characters should not be surprised if they suffer from a stress-related disease, whether IBS or something else. Even though their basic personalities are determined genetically and reinforced through childhood, adolescence, and beyond, they can still learn techniques to cope with stress, whether that stress is hurled outward at other people or pushed inward. Both can be equally destructive.

In between these two types is the person who is a mixture of the other two—inwardly fairly angry but outwardly passive. She conceals her feelings, bottles up her anger, and is then surprised that she develops a stress-related condition. But IBS is very common among people who appear to be unemotional, organized, and in control. They are often quite set in their ways and don't like change. They turn their stress inward like the passive person, rather than outward like the aggressive person.

## Vulnerability: Passiveness and Low Self-Esteem

Vulnerable people tend to have many of these characteristics:

—Saying yes when they want to say no

—Not refusing other people's requests

—Not expressing their feelings easily

—Bottling things up

—Feeling taken advantage of

—Being anxious and easily depressed

—Worrying

—Being sensitive and easily hurt

—Erecting an invisible wall around them to keep out the world's problems

—Lacking confidence

—Working in a boring, unchallenging job

—Having difficulty relaxing

—Lacking energy

—Dwelling on negative things and expecting the worst

—Being indecisive

—Not feeling in control of their life or health

Despite this list of apparently negative qualities, people like this tend to be well-liked by friends and colleagues, are easy to get along with, can be good friends to others, and are always willing to help. So if you feel you are a passive, vulnerable person, don't have a low opinion of yourself because you are not outgoing and aggressive—your qualities are much valued. People are not judging you as harshly as you judge yourself—quite the opposite. You are almost certainly a much-valued friend and colleague.

Perhaps you wish you were more attractive, sophisticated, clever, bold, forceful, and dynamic. Maybe you are waiting for some future time when everything will be different—when you are richer, more successful, married, have children, or free from the children—in fact, you find it quite hard to enjoy the here-and-now. This is where self-talk can be so powerful, both positively and negatively. Self-talk is those things we say to ourselves:

"I'm not as attractive as she is."

"Nothing ever goes right for me."

"It's all so unfair."

"I knew I should have said no."

"I can't help how I feel."

"I must put other people's needs before my own."

"I mustn't show I'm feeling upset and angry."

"I'm like this because it runs in the family."

"How can people treat me like this?"

And so on, on and on. You can probably think of many more that are directly relevant to you. But you needn't say these sorts of things to yourself. Each time your self-talk niggles away at your self-esteem, think up a positive statement that is the opposite of what you were thinking. Repeat it several times a day, and gradually you will "accentuate the positive, eliminate the negative." Here are some possible examples:

"People at work like me."

"I can make things happen the way I want them to."

"Even if something upsets me, I can make sure I do not remain upset for long."

"I can learn to change how I feel and respond to situations; I do not have to let them worry me."

"I can accept myself for what I am."

"I have the right to express how I feel."

"Everyone makes mistakes sometimes; I don't make any more mistakes than other people do."

"Lots of things about me are very attractive and likable."

"Losers let it happen; winners make it happen."

These are just some examples of how the things you say to yourself can affect how you feel. When your self-esteem is high, you will feel less vulnerable and vice versa. Your self-esteem is your evaluation of yourself, and you should use all your self-talk and positive thinking to keep that evaluation high. If you place a high value on being slim, successful in business, good at tennis, or successful at raising children, and you are none of these, then your self-esteem will suffer. Try to reorder your priorities so that what you are good at is important to you; there are things about you that people like and envy, so build on them to keep your self-esteem high.

From now on give yourself permission to

—Change your mind

—Express your feelings

—Say no when you want to

—Be the person you are

—Distance yourself from other people's problems

—Have needs and wants

—Make mistakes

—Be the judge of your own actions

—Not have any reason to do all these things

# Aggressiveness

Aggressive people are not good for themselves nor for those they live and work with. Aggression increases your blood pressure, your risk of coronary heart disease, your level of stress, your risk of accidents, and your chance of getting a stress-related condition. It contributes to marriage breakdown, domestic stress, alcoholism, discord at work, violence, road accidents, and much, much more.

In the early 1970s, Friedman and Rosenman studied over 3,400 men who had suffered from coronary heart disease. At least 85 percent of them had a personality type that the two researchers called Type A. The results of their research were published in a book called *Type A Behavior and Your Heart*, which should be compulsory reading for all those who want to ensure that their aggressive personality doesn't lead them to an early grave. Since many sufferers of IBS have this type of personality it could also have been called *Type A Behavior and Your Irritable Bowel!*

Type A (aggressive) people have many of these characteristics:

—Hostility

—Competitiveness

—Quarrelsomeness

—Restlessness

—Impatience

—Frivolous talking

—Frequent swearing

—Constant feeling of time pressure

—Ambition

—Preoccupation with deadlines

—Hypersensitivity to criticism

—Inability to delegate for fear of losing control

—Obsessive punctuality

—Contempt of those who are slow or inadequate performers

—Continually creating new goals and seldom achieving old ones

—Believing they work more effectively under pressure

—Dominating conversations

—Holding stereotyped generalizations about groups

—Striving for achievement

Do many of these characteristics describe you? If so, don't ignore it. Type A behavior is taken as a serious risk factor for disease, about which something can and should be done. Type A people (who are much more likely to be men than women) meet in groups to help each other. They are taught to modify their behavior, which improves their relationships with other people and reduces their high risk of heart attack. Members of the group discuss how they have reacted to particular situations, and they work out how they could have reacted better, without impatience or anger, so that next time they will handle the situation more skillfully.

If you are a Type A person, there are many things about you that people like: you are self-assured, efficient, enthusiastic, and interesting; and these are qualities worth building on. But if you can be aware of those other characteristics that people may not like and try to control those qualities, you could have the best of all worlds. Most people prefer people who are pleasant, friendly, accepting, helpful, cooperative, open, relaxed, and warm.

You too could be like this. You may feel you don't want to lose your competitive edge or feel so calm you don't get things done on time. You don't need to. You can simply learn to be less Type A without going too far the other way. Like the vulnerable, passive people, you probably engage in self-talk too, and it could be reinforcing your basic aggressive personality:

"I am very ambitious."

"I drive myself hard."

"I can't stand incompetence and inefficiency."

"I need to win to prove what I am."

"Making mistakes is a sign of weakness. So is admitting that you don't know something."

"Showing affection is only for wimps."

"The job will be done much better if I do it myself."

"Using strong language means I am strong."

And so on. Yet by changing those things you say to yourself, you could become less Type A while still retaining your strengths:

"Because I am a strong person, I can afford to show affection."

"Everyone makes mistakes, and no one will think less of me if I do so too."

"Delegating a job is the sign of a responsible manager."

"I don't need to prove I am strong."

"If someone does a job slower than I do, I can accept that calmly."

"It's OK to be gentle, slow, wrong, last. . . ."

"I can admit my mistakes."

"I can learn from other people."

"If I get something wrong, I will not be a failure."

"Waiting is a *gift* of time, not a *waste* of time."

Give yourself permission to

—Be wrong

—Ask for help

—Hug someone

—Do a job slowly

—Be late

—Cry

—Come in second, or even last

—Remain silent

—Enjoy birds singing, water flowing, children playing

—Fail

—Feel frightened

—Let other people make decisions

—Drive slowly

—Relax

In their book, Friedman and Rosenman say, "If you are overly hostile, certainly the most important drill measure you should adopt is that one in which you remind yourself of the fact that you are hostile." And having done that, resolve to do things differently! Modifying your behavior won't make you a wimp or boring, because your basic interesting personality is still there. But it may make life calmer and less stressful for your family and workmates, and it should reduce your chances of getting coronary heart disease and help alleviate your IBS.

## Assertiveness: The Right Balance

Imagine these two situations:

Your friend tells you she has had the offer of a job, but she wouldn't get home until about 6:00 p.m., and she has come to ask you if you would be able to collect her son from school every day and keep him with you until she gets home. She says there's no one else she could ask, and if you can't have her son she will have to turn down the job. You greatly value her friendship, but you really don't want to be committed to having him every day after school.

If you say no, you risk losing a friendship that is important to you, but if you say yes, you will probably resent the commitment involved and feel annoyed with your friend for asking you and with yourself for agreeing to do it.

You are involved in a minor road collision with another driver, and both cars receive some damage. You think it's his fault, he thinks it's yours. He is angry, aggressive, and personally insulting about your driving. Do you shout back at him, giving as good as you get, his aggression matched only by yours? Or do you take his insults without retaliating and then when you get home feel indescribably angry that he should have been so aggressive and that you let him get away with it?

Both these situations are likely to get your irritable bowel working overtime, but there is a solution that can help you, your friend, the other driver, and your gut. It's called assertiveness.

A few years ago, a group that I belonged to decided to take a course in assertiveness training. I didn't know what it was, and I wasn't particularly interested, but since everyone else had signed up for it, I decided to follow the crowd. It turned out to be one of the most valuable things I have ever done. Like so many people, I often wished I had been able to express myself differently on a particular occasion—perhaps more positively, perhaps less aggressively. Assertiveness training taught me how to do it. I don't get it right every time, but there are now fewer occasions when I feel I have said yes when I wanted to say no or antagonized someone by using inappropriate words.

There have probably been many occasions when you knew you used the wrong words or the wrong tone of voice or chose the wrong time to say something; when you felt you didn't have a full opportunity to say how you felt; when you felt unable to express how you felt; when you were afraid of provoking a wrong reaction in someone else; when you expected that person to respond in one way and he or she responded quite differently. From all these situations you may come away hurt, bruised, angry, or frustrated, yet not know how to make sure it doesn't happen again. In fact, the more hurt and angry you are the harder it becomes to use an understanding tone of voice or considerate words.

The person who uses an aggressive manner puts his wants, needs, and rights above those of other people. He tries to get his own way by not allowing others a choice. His behavior may be active or passive, direct or indirect, honest or dishonest, but it always communicates the appearance of superiority. He wins, others lose—which can all too easily lead to a situation where others want to get their own back.

At the opposite extreme is behavior that communicates a message of inferiority, the person who always gives in to others, the doormat, the victim. She allows the wants, needs, and rights of other people to be more important than her own. Others win, she loses.

But there is a middle way—assertiveness. The assertive person communicates respect for himself and others. His wants, needs, and rights are equal to other people's. He will influence, listen, and negotiate in a way that causes others to cooperate willingly, with no desire to retaliate. With assertiveness, both sides "win."

As you may now see, assertiveness is not aggressiveness. It is not dominating other people, nor being dominated. It is not being unfeminine, unmasculine, overbearing, ruthless, or hostile. There is a tendency for men to think they should be aggressive and for women to think they should not—both these assumptions often cause conflict. An assertive woman is not an aggressive woman. She may get her own way or she may allow others to have their own way, but it will be a win-win situation, not one side winning while the other side loses.

This book is about Irritable Bowel Syndrome and stress, and it is not possible here to teach assertiveness. But it is a skill almost everyone can benefit from. In many areas classes are held to teach the technique, often in all-female or all-male groups, so that the environment is relaxed and nonthreatening. Subjects that might be covered in an assertiveness course may include:

—Making requests

—Saying no to other people's requests and feeling all right about it

—Giving criticism and compliments

—Receiving criticism and compliments

—Expressing your own anger

—Handling other people's anger

—Using body language appropriately

—Developing self-confidence and self-esteem

—Resolving conflicts

—Being assertive with your own children

If you are unable to find a group, there are two very useful books you could read: *When I Say No I Feel Guilty*, by Manuel J. Smith, and *A Woman in Your Own Right—Assertiveness and You*, by Anne Dickson. If you have never thought about assertiveness before, it will open up to you a whole new way of responding to other people that will benefit you for the rest of your life.

## Learning to Relax

Imagine you are holding a lemon. Now, in your mind, cut it in quarters and suck out the juice of a whole quarter. Feel the juice on your lips and tongue, notice its sharpness. Did anything happen? You probably noticed saliva coming into your mouth and your tongue reacting as if you really had felt the sharp tang of the lemon.

This is a simple example of how the activities of the mind affect the responses in the body. In Irritable Bowel Syndrome, the effect can be just as noticeable: You feel tense and anxious, and your intestines start going into spasm; you relax, and they calm down again. Perhaps one day researchers will identify the exact process by which this happens and develop a reliable treatment, but until then the best thing you can do for yourself is to remain as calm as possible and avoid the sort of situations that provoke your intestines and make your life uncomfortable.

This chapter suggests several ways in which you can put the busy world to one side for a while and just *r-e-l-a-x*. If you do not already make regular times for yourself to do nothing special, this may not seem an easy or proper thing to do. From childhood we are encouraged to fill each moment with something worthwhile; doing nothing is "lazy." Some children were even taught to believe it is sinful. So we grow up unable to truly relax and feeling guilty if we take time out for ourselves. How often have you sat quietly reading the paper or watching television or just putting your feet up, when your neighbor drops in? What do you do? The chances are that you apologize—"I'm sorry, I was just sitting down for a moment while the teapot boiled/ the paint dried. . . ." and so on. The implication is that normally you would be filling each moment with something wonderfully useful and that you feel slightly guilty to be discovered doing something such as putting your feet up for a few minutes.

In case these sort of feelings worry you, start by taking out only a few minutes each day for relaxing. Keep it short, just long enough to start feeling quiet inside yourself. Some very tense people find it extremely difficult to let go, and this is where allowing yourself to relax is much more effective than making yourself relax. Relaxation is about "not doing," and this is what so many people find difficult. So try to put aside those exhortations from childhood and give yourself permission to be "not doing." You may have a lot of things to do, but however busy you are you can still spare a few minutes to sit quietly and empty your mind of the pressures of the moment.

Learning to relax and let go has many benefits:

—Control over your life

—An enhanced sense of well-being

—More positive feelings about yourself and your capabilities

—Less anxiety and more confidence

—The ability to put stress in perspective

—Improved sleep

—A quieter digestive system

—A reduction in other stress-related conditions

—Less fatigue

—The ability to calm someone else who is upset or anxious

With a relaxation program, you are in control. You are choosing to do it, and you can stop any time you want to. You can do as much or as little as you choose, when you choose, how you choose. You choose the position, the time, the place, and the exercises that suit you best; when you have had enough, you choose to stop.

Any of the following activities can help you to relax:

—Buy a cassette tape or CD of relaxation or "mood music." You can find these at record shops or health food stores, or look at the advertisements in magazines.

—Drink a relaxing herb tea. Try one containing chamomile or valerian.

—Have a warm (not too hot) bath, with soothing additives such as chamomile, valerian, or sandalwood oil.

—Sit in a chair in front of a long mirror. How do you look? Tense or relaxed? Are you sitting on the edge of the chair or comfortably back into it? What are your hands doing? Practice sitting in a way that, seen in the mirror, looks relaxed and at peace. Then remember this practice every time you sit in a chair. This will help you to see yourself as you would like others to see you.

—As you go about the house, stop and, without changing your facial expression, look at yourself in the mirror. What do you see? What do others see? A frown, a tight mouth, or a calm, pleasant facial expression? Relax your face and smile at yourself in the mirror.

It is true that you cannot have a relaxed body with a tense mind, so obviously you must calm your mind before you can calm your body. But you can put the cart before the horse somewhat. By relaxing your body you can indeed start to relax your mind. So make sure that each part of you is without tension and outwardly still, and you will be a long way toward making yourself inwardly still.

In addition, there are certain exercises you can do for muscle relaxation and proper breathing. Some exercises will work for you and perhaps some won't; some may not work at first but will after a while. So try any that appeal to you and come back to others later if you want to. While you are doing any form of relaxation, suspend all value judgements and intellectual criticism. And when you have finished, avoid the tendency to say to yourself, "Well, I've done my relaxation for today," and then rush around as tense and stressed out as ever, undoing all the good you have achieved.

## Setting Yourself Up for Relaxation

Relaxation needs no special equipment, no skilled teacher, and no drugs. You can do it almost anywhere. It is simple, and it works.

What you do need is commitment to doing it, a reasonably quiet environment, a comfortable position, and an open, receptive attitude. If you can put aside a regular time each day it will be more effective, but even if you can't, you will still benefit.

### Where?

A quiet, warm, comfortable place is the ideal, but anywhere is better than nowhere. Try to be undisturbed by people or the telephone. Because you can relax lying or sitting, you will need either some floor space or an upright or easy chair, or a sofa or meditation cushion—whatever is convenient and comfortable.

### When?

The best time is when you know you can put aside a few minutes and will be undisturbed. It may be first thing in the morning, during the lunch break, after work, during the afternoon, or at bedtime. Try different times and see which works best for you. Right after meals is not the best time for most people (because digestion seems to interfere with relaxation), but it may be just right for you. At least to begin with, you may settle down more quickly if you can choose the same time and place each day, so that you come to associate that time and place with being relaxed.

### For How Long?

Once you are doing some form of relaxation regularly each day or so, you will probably be taking somewhere between fifteen and thirty minutes. It may be all at one time or in two separate sessions, but the greatest gains will come if you can do it regularly. If you are saying to yourself, "Where am I going to find an extra thirty minutes a day? I'm far too busy already," then that just demonstrates your need to relax. The time to relax is when you have no time to relax! If time is a problem to you, start with just five minutes once or twice a day, and build up when you feel able to—but do try to do at least something every day.

### What Do I Wear?

What you wear is up to you. Whatever you are wearing right now will do—or something completely different. If possible, have clothing that is loose around the neck and waist, but if you have no choice but to do relaxation exercises in a suit and tie, then just loosen anything that feels tight. If possible, take off your shoes and eyeglasses (if you wear them).

### What Position Should I Be In?

However you are most comfortable. Here are some ideas:

—Sit on an upright chair with your spine straight. Keep your head easily balanced on your neck, with your chin pointing slightly down rather than slightly up. Imagine you are being pulled up like a puppet by a thread attached to the crown of your head (the crown is considerably farther back than the forehead). Place your feet flat on the floor, legs slightly apart, hands resting comfortably on your lap, palms facing up or down, whichever you prefer. If your feet don't touch the floor, rest them on a book or something similar. Keep your body equally balanced between the left and right side, rather than putting your weight and balance mainly on to one side. Move around until you feel symmetrical. Shut your eyes.

—Sit in an easy chair, with your back resting comfortably against the back of the chair. A small cushion in the small of your back may give you more spinal support. Place your feet flat on the floor, a comfortable distance apart, and rest your hands on your lap, palms facing up or down. Shut your eyes.

—Sit on a meditation stool or cushion with your spine straight, head pulled up from the crown, hands on your lap, and eyes closed.

—Lie on a sofa, with your body in a straight line, not twisted to one side or the other. Your legs should be about shoulder-width apart, feet flopping outward. Your hands can be by your side or on your abdomen, palms facing up or down. You may be more comfortable if you put a small cushion or pillow under your head, behind your knees, in the small of your back. Shut your eyes.

—Lie on the floor on a thick blanket, in the same position as on a sofa.

These are all comfortable positions, ideal for relaxing. But the idea isn't to go to sleep but rather to achieve deep relaxation while you are still awake (unless you are relaxing specifically to help insomnia).

### *How Do I Finish?*

When you have done as much as you want to, just remain where you are for a minute or two with your eyes closed, breathing quietly. Then open your eyes and bring your mind back to the room you are in. Stretch your body from your heels to the top of your head and, if you are lying down, turn on to your side for a while. Then when you are ready, get up slowly. Don't rush off in a stressful, hectic manner, since this will negate what you have done; instead, get up quietly and try to maintain a feeling of calm for as long as possible.

Now try the following exercises. At first nothing may seem to happen, you may be disappointed and feel this is for other people but not for you. But don't be discouraged, because regular relaxation will be helping you even if you are unaware of it. Some people give up when they don't see instant results, but this is a pity, because benefits begin before you are aware of any improvement.

## Exercises for Relaxation

There are numerous books available on how to relax, and your library or bookshop will probably have several. Included here is a collection of different forms of relaxation exercises, so you can choose which suits you best.

MUSCLE-RELAXATION EXERCISES

*Exercise One:* Let your breath out, then breath in, then do a long out-breath. Continue to breathe calmly while you lower your shoulders, relax your neck, and unclench your jaw and your hands. Try to keep your voice low and calm. Visualize your digestive system remaining calm and peaceful. Say to yourself, "I am in control of this situation."

*Exercise Two:* Examine each part of your body in turn and see if any set of muscles is tense. Work upwards from your toes to your head, thinking about each bit of you: your right foot, right leg, left foot, left leg—are they quite relaxed? Then your right hand, right arm, left hand, left arm—is there any tension there, particularly in your fingers? Now your abdomen—the source of your Irritable Bowel Syndrome. Feel it being quite calm and relaxed, no tension, no spasm, just rising and falling gently as you breathe. Next your shoulders and neck, relaxed and heavy. Finally your jaw, mouth, eyes, forehead—no tension at all here, quite slack.

Tense people block out signs of tense muscles, so they become less aware of stress within themselves. A simple exercise like this encourages you to be aware of tension in yourself and so overcome it. As you notice any tense muscles, concentrate more on relaxing that set.

*Exercise Three:* To relax your shoulders, sit upright on a chair, hands relaxed in your lap and with your back straight but not stiff. Breathe in and as you do so, raise your shoulders toward your ears. Hold for a count of five, then slowly release your breath and lower your shoulders. Repeat a few times. This is a good exercise to do when you are stuck in a traffic jam.

*Exercise Four:* Sit or lie in a comfortable position. Close your eyes and become aware of your breathing. Each time you exhale, notice a different part of your body in turn and feel it being physically supported by the chair, sofa, or floor. Become very aware of that part of you on each outbreath and feel the heaviness of it. As you concentrate on it, say "My [part of the body] is warm and soft and heavy." Imagine that part sinking deeply into the floor or the sofa, so heavy that you couldn't possibly lift it up. Continue upward until each part of you feels beautifully warm and soft and heavy.

*Exercise Five:* Having relaxed all your muscles in turn, you could now go one step further and consciously tense them up. Once again, sit or lie in a comfortable position and, starting with your feet, tense each set of muscles, then tense them even harder, then relax them. This tension will bring even greater relaxation. However, don't tense your abdominal muscles—they tense up all too easily, and any extra tension might make them worse.

## BREATHING EXERCISES

Breathing exercises are one of the easiest ways to achieve a feeling of calm, and they have the advantage that you can do them anywhere, at any time. They have the apparently contradictory effect of giving you energy when you feel tired and calming you down when you feel tense. So next time you feel the need for a cup of coffee, a cigarette, or a strong drink, just do breathing exercises for a minute or two instead—it's much better for your IBS.

When you are calm and relaxed, you breathe from the diaphragm. Look at someone sleeping on her back and you will see a gentle rising and falling movement from the area below the ribs. When you are tense, you breathe from high up in your chest. So a quiet state of mind produces breathing from the diaphragm; but you can also put the cart before the horse and induce a state of calm by breathing from that place.

There is also another advantage in this level of breathing: the diaphragm is a strong sheet of muscle that separates the chest cavity from the abdomen, and as it contracts during breathing, it pushes the abdominal organs downward and forward, gently compressing and massaging them. So by doing breathing exercises regularly you benefit both your mind and your abdomen.

While you are doing the exercises, concentrate on your breath and try not to let other thoughts come into your mind. If they do, don't get bothered or distracted by them—simply put those thoughts to one side for the moment and return your mind to your breath.

A word about breathing exercises: Sometimes this form of relaxation may bring to the surface of your mind thoughts and feelings that have been buried for a long time, and these thoughts may upset you. If this happens, be aware of them, accept them, and try not to become upset by them. Most thoughts of this kind are better out then in, but if they distress you, just stretch, open your eyes, and come out of the exercise. You are in charge, you can stop at any time.

Breathing exercises can increase the level of oxygen in the blood to a point at which you feel lightheaded or your fingers begin to tingle. If this happens, just breathe in a panting shallow way for a few moments, to reduce your oxygen level. As with any unhelpful thoughts, you can stop any time you choose by coming out of the exercise.

***Exercise Six:*** Start by doing an exercise lying on your back, with your feet a comfortable distance apart, and a sense of balance between the left and right sides of your body; move until you feel quite symmetrical. Place your hands in the area of your abdomen just below your rIBS and breathe from deep down so you feel that area rising and falling under your hands. Then, keeping your hands over your abdomen, breathe from high up in your chest so that you hardly feel your hands moving at all but are aware of your shoulders moving slightly. Finally, return to quiet abdominal breathing for a few minutes, just noticing the rise and fall of your hands. When you are ready, get up slowly.

***Exercise Seven:*** Lie as for Exercise Six, but place one hand on your abdomen as before and one hand on your chest. As you breathe, notice which hand is moving and by how much. Concentrate on the rise and fall of your hands. Then with the next breath, be aware of the air filling up from the diaphragm to the chest, of your lower hand moving before your upper one. Do this for a few minutes, all the time being aware of the air coming in through your nostrils, filling your lungs from the bottom up and then emptying out again. Try to think of nothing but your breath coming in and out.

***Exercise Eight:*** These next set of exercises can be done sitting or lying down. Find a comfortable position, shut your eyes, and be aware of your outbreath. Notice how, after an outbreath, the inbreath just seems to happen. Again, do a long outbreath. Repeat several times: long outbreath followed by a short inbreath, concentrating particularly on the outbreath.

*Exercise Nine:* This time, instead of noticing inbreaths separate from outbreaths, see them as one complete circular movement in which each leads on from the other with no perceptible difference between them.

*Exercise Ten:* First, breathe out deeply to expel stale air. Then breathe in slowly and deeply to a count of two. Next, hold your breath for a count of four. Finally, breathe out for a count of four. So it's in two, hold four, out four. Do this for two or three minutes, but stop if you feel dizzy. All the while, concentrate on the breath.

*Exercise Eleven* (alternate nostril breathing): First, identify your fingers—working outward from the thumb they are the thumb, index finger, middle finger, ring finger, little finger. Next, sit with your spine straight, eyes shut, and your whole body relaxed. If you wear eyeglasses, it is best to remove them. Place the index and middle fingers of your right hand on the bridge of your nose between your eyebrows. With the ring finger of your right hand close the left nostril. (If you are left-handed, you may prefer to reverse the instructions.) Breathe out through your right nostril, then breathe in through the same (right) nostril. Lift your ring finger slightly, close your right nostril with your thumb, and breathe out through your left nostril, then in through the same (left) nostril. Lift your thumb slightly and repeat from this sequence for several minutes, remembering to breathe out first through each nostril. Listen to your breathing. Concentrate on it. If your mind wanders, be aware of this and bring it gently back.

Although this exercise seems complicated to describe, it is a simple, soothing rhythm once you see how to do it. Gentle pressure on the nostrils is thought to relieve menstrual cramps, so there is a possibility that it might relieve abdominal cramps, too.

*Exercise Twelve:* Get into a comfortable position. Relax all your muscles and feel your body being supported by whatever you are sitting or lying on. Breathe naturally—notice the cool breath coming in through your nostrils and the warm air going out again. Be aware of this for a few minutes. Now, as you breathe out, visualize in any way that is comfortable to you the air carrying out from your body all the pain and tension that is inside you. Each breath takes away more pain and tension, and with successive breaths your whole abdominal area becomes relaxed and comfortable. When you are ready, stretch from your heels to the top of your head, open your eyes, and gently get up.

**Exercise Thirteen:** The most effective way to do this exercise is to record it on tape and play it back when you want to relax. Read it into the microphone using a slow calm voice; pause for a moment at the end of each phrase. If you are not happy with the first recording, make a note of any changes you need to make and do it again.

Begin by breathing out first. Then breathe in easily, just as much as you need. Now breathe out slowly, with a slight sigh like a balloon slowly deflating. Do this once more, slowly. Breathe in, breathe out . . . . As you breathe out, feel the tension begin to drain away. Then go back to your ordinary breathing—even, quiet, steady. Now direct your thoughts in turn to each part of your body.

Think first about your left foot. Your toes are still. Your foot feels heavy on the floor. Let your foot and toes start to feel completely relaxed. Now think about your right foot . . . toes . . . ankles . . . they are resting heavily on the floor. Let both your feet, your toes, ankles start to relax.

Now think about your legs. Let your legs feel completely relaxed and heavy on the chair. Your thighs, your knees roll outward when they relax, so let them go.

Think now about your back and your spine. Let the tension drain away from your back and from your spine. Notice your breathing—each time you breathe out, relax your back and spine a little more.

Let your abdominal muscles become soft and loose. There's no need to hold your stomach in tight. It rises and falls as you breathe quietly. Feel your stomach completely relax.

No tension in your chest. Let your breathing be slow and easy. Each time you breathe out, let go a little more.

Think now about the fingers of your left hand—they are curved, limp, and quite still. Now the fingers of your right hand . . . relaxed . . . soft and still. Let this feeling of relaxation spread—up to your arms . . . Feel the heaviness in your arms up to your shoulders. . . . Let your shoulders relax, let them drop easily . . . and then let them drop even further than you thought they could.

Think about your neck. Feel the tension melt away from your neck and shoulders. Each time you breathe out, relax your neck a little more.

Now, before going any further, just check to see if all these parts of your body are still relaxed—your feet, legs, back and spine, tummy, hands, arms, neck, and shoulders. Keep your breathing gentle and easy. Every time you breathe out, relax a little more and let all the tensions ease away from your body. No tensions . . . just enjoy this feeling of relaxation.

Now think about your face. Let the expression come off your face. Smooth out your brow and let your forehead feel wide and relaxed. Let your eyebrows drop gently. There's no tension around your eyes . . . your eyelids slightly closed, your eyes are still. Let your jaw unwind . . . teeth slightly apart as your jaw unwinds more and more.

Feel the relief of letting go.

Now think about your tongue and throat. Let your tongue drop down to the bottom of your mouth and relax completely. Relax your tongue and throat. And your lips . . . lightly together, no pressure between them.

Let all the muscles in your face unwind and let go—there's no tension in your face . . . just let it relax more and more.

Now, instead of thinking about yourself in parts, feel the all-over sensation of letting go, of quiet and of rest. Check to see if you are still relaxed. Stay like this for a few moments and listen to your breathing . . . in . . . and out. . . . Let your body become looser, heavier, each time you breathe out.

Now continue for a little longer and enjoy this time for relaxation.

Finally, wriggle your hands and your feet a little. When you are ready, open your eyes and sit quietly for a while. Stretch . . . then slowly start to move again. (This is reproduced from the Workers' Educational Association pack on Women and Health, with permission of the Health Education Authority.)

Practice some form of relaxation every day—in the car, at a computer, at the sink, ironing board, workbench, desk . . . wherever you are. Just pause, take a deep breath, and consciously relax your muscles. Once you have practiced being relaxed in a calm place on your own, you will be able to be relaxed at other times: in a meeting, during discussions, while driving or shopping, doing household jobs, when you are bored or frustrated, and even when your spouse or children drive you mad. Having developed the habit of relaxation, it will come quite naturally to you.

In the beginning, when you have achieved a state of peacefulness even for a few minutes, take time to mentally record the experience. Recall what you did and how you felt and remember yourself in that situation being relaxed. This will reinforce your expectation of being relaxed, and relaxation will get progressively easier.

As you go through the day, notice how you are standing or sitting. If you are standing with your weight on one leg, move until both feet are carrying equal weight. When you sit with your legs crossed, become aware of it and place both feet flat on the floor with your legs relaxed. (If, like me, you are fairly short, this is easier said than done, as most chairs seem to be designed for tall people with long legs!) Are your shoulders tense? Then lower them, feel your neck stretching out, your muscles relaxed. Are you tapping your fingers, banging your knees, clenching your teeth, jingling the coins in your pocket? Notice it, then just relax those tense muscles. Get into the habit of noticing these little things and making changes. The buildup of tension in your muscles is a sign of your tense mind; by relaxing muscles that you can see and control, you will be aware of the general tension in your body that is also present in your abdomen. You have no direct control over the muscles of the colon, but the tension within you affects the way those muscles propel food. Reducing your overall level of stress and tension will indirectly cause those muscles to relax.

## Meditation and Yoga

Mantras, joss sticks, and headstands—is this your image of meditation and yoga? Eastern nonsense? All very well for people who like that kind of thing but not for you?

Mantras are words said repetitively to help concentrate the mind and direct it away from the present. In your life you may achieve a similar effect by concentrating so hard on something that the effort becomes quite relaxing.

Standing on your head is a form of exercise that also takes up all your concentration and leaves you feeling relaxed and invigorated. You may be getting exercise that has a similar effect.

So these disciplines are perhaps not as wildly different from what you already do. But meditation and yoga can achieve other benefits that most ordinary forms of exercise can't. Regularly practicing either of these can lower your heartbeat and blood pressure, improve your sleep, decrease anxiety, increase alertness, heighten your concentration ability and your general well-being, and bring a feeling of calm and release from tension.

People who practice meditation regularly tend to be less anxious than others and recover quicker after stressful incidents.

## Meditation

As with all relaxation exercises, meditation can be done anywhere but is more beneficial if you can choose a time and place where you will be comfortable and undisturbed. It is important to divert your mind from your normal thought processes. Suspend all judgment and intellectual criticism. Just be patient and open, and in time you will be pleased at the changes you start to notice, both in your mind and, hopefully, in your irritable bowel.

Meditation, like breathing exercises, can sometimes bring thoughts to the surface of your mind that make you feel agitated or anxious. This is quite normal. If this happens, simply open your eyes, have a good stretch, and come out of the exercise. As before, you are in control, you can stop when you want to.

## MEDITATION EXERCISES

*Exercise One:* As with the breathing exercises, sit or lie in a comfortable position. Mentally scan your whole body and consciously relax all your muscles from your feet up to your head. Concentrate particularly on whatever part of your body you often tense up. Breathe normally. When you feel quite relaxed, as you breathe out say the word "one" either out loud or to yourself. Then breathe in normally. Continue like this, saying "one" each time you breathe out. Try to concentrate on the normal breathing and the word "one." Your mind will probably wander; if it does just be aware of this and bring your thoughts gently back to the word "one." After about ten minutes, continue normal breathing without saying "one," just being quiet, with your eyes closed. Then open your eyes, take in the room around you, and when you are ready get up. If you prefer, you could say "peace" instead, or any word that seems right for you. After each exercise, don't worry whether you have successfully achieved what you believe meditation to be. In time it will come.

*Exercise Two:* This is an exercise in noticing yourself. As you sit quietly, notice your internal feelings: your breathing, any digestive rumbles, your closed eyelids on your eyeballs, your tongue in your mouth, your heart beating, your hands and feet resting against the floor or against a part of your body. Then notice other body feelings: your toes in your socks and shoes, the waistband of your trousers or skirt, your neckband or tie, your cuffs around your wrists, how your clothes feel on your skin. Finally, notice external sounds: cars going by, dogs barking, someone walking past, people talking, any smells in the air. Identify each thing, but do not allow yourself to think about it or get distracted by it. Repeat this from the beginning as many times as you want to.

*Exercise Three:* Place a lighted candle a few feet in front of you. Concentrate on it until you feel you can't look at it any longer. Then shut your eyes and you will see the afterimage of the candle and the flame in front of you. Concentrate on this afterimage until it fades from your mind. Then open your eyes and look at the real candle again. Repeat this as many times as you want to.

*Exercise Four:* Create in your mind an image of your troublesome gut (or any other part that's bothering you). How you see it can be abstract, symbolic, or anatomically correct—it doesn't matter. Just hold the picture in your mind. Now imagine your body's defense mechanisms (again this can be abstract or symbolic or anatomically correct) moving to your gut, soothing it, calming it. Let your imagination run wild: see your gut responding, see any spasms dying down, any muscular contortions fading away. Now your gut is pain free and propelling food in a smooth, gentle way— up the right side of your abdomen, across the middle, and down the left side, like a river flowing. Visualize yourself going about your life with your bowel made pain free by your body's natural mechanisms. Then open your eyes, observe the room you are in, take a few breaths, stretch, and get up slowly.

*Exercise Five:* As you breathe normally, focus your thoughts on the rise and fall of your abdomen and of the air flowing in and out of your nostrils. As you breathe in count 1, and as you breathe out count 2, in count 3, out count 4, and so on up to 10. Then start again: in 1, out 2, in 3, out 4. . . . Don't attempt to control or manipulate your breath. Just let it happen naturally, being aware of it. Continue doing this as long as you want to, trying to keep your mind on nothing but your breathing.

*Exercise Six:* Hold five beads or pebbles in one hand. Pass them slowly one at a time to the other hand. Feel each one, count it, hear the sound it makes against the others. Pass the beads from one hand to the other as many times as you want to, focusing your attention on the beads, thinking of nothing else apart from them, their sound and feel.

*Exercise Seven:* This is a useful exercise if something is troubling you and preventing you from directing your mind to other things. Sit comfortably, breathing quietly. Now focus on whatever is disturbing you but don't get caught up in it. Don't allow yourself to wallow in worrying thoughts. Try to give a shape to this problem—any shape you like—until it is an actual object, not just a thought. Now imagine you are standing back from this object that is your worry and looking at it objectively. In your imagination, put the shape into a box. Imagine getting wrapping paper and cellophane tape and scissors and imagine using the scissors to cut out some wrapping paper, wrap it around the box, and secure it with tape. Let yourself be really imaginative about this. When the shape is nicely wrapped up in the box, take the box and put it somewhere safe where you can't see it while you get on with your life, but where it will be when you need to face up to it again. Now see yourself getting on with your life with this particular problem out of the way. You can leave it there as long as you choose to, but at some time you will need to come back to it, to unwrap it, and face it, although all the time you know you can put it back in its box when you want to. End the session by returning your thoughts to where you are at present, in the room you are in. As before, take a few deep breaths, stretch, and get up when you feel ready.

*Exercise Eight:* Record the following on tape, in a slow, calm voice, pausing slightly after each phrase:

Imagine yourself walking out of the room you are in. You go outside and see a magic carpet there. You get on to the carpet and make yourself comfortable. You are going to fly right away from here to somewhere tropical. You are flying above towns and villages, fields and farms. The houses and cars look unreal, like matchbox toys. Now you are over a beach and now over the sea. At first the sea is gray, but as you get to a warmer climate it gets bluer and bluer. You can feel the sun beating down on you, warming you up. Ahead you see a lush island with palm trees, white sands, and clear blue sea. You land on the beach and look around you for a minute or two, breathing in the richly scented warm air. You take a stroll on the beach barefoot and feel the warmth of the sand on the soles of your feet. Dip your toes in the sea; it feels cool and refreshing. Now walk into the jungle. There are beautiful exotic flowers everywhere—they smell wonderful and have clear bright colors: pinks, yellows, turquoise. High above you are monkeys, jumping from tree to tree chattering to each other; there are also parrots flying around. Ahead you see a clearing through the trees and you walk toward it. There is a sleepy green lagoon bathed in green light from the sun passing through the tallest palm trees. On the lagoon is a little dinghy; you get into it and lie down.

You are bobbing gently in the lagoon in a pool of green light. You can hear the monkeys and birds in the jungle, but they sound a long way off. You can smell the fragrance of the exotic flowers and fruits. Just enough sun can get through the trees to warm your body as you lie on the dinghy. Let yourself completely unwind as you relax, taking in the warmth and smells and sounds of the jungle.

When you are ready to come back, get up from the dinghy and walk slowly back through the jungle to your magic carpet. Make yourself comfortable on the carpet again for your journey home. You are flying over the sea, then over land, and now you can see your home town. You land back where you started from and walk back into the room.

(This exercise is reproduced from the *Workers' Educational Association pack on Women and Health,* with permission of the Health Education Authority.)

# Yoga

All these meditation exercises have involved nothing more strenuous than sitting in a chair or lying on the floor. Yoga postures are slightly more active. The best way to do yoga really is to join a class with a qualified instructor who will teach you to do the postures correctly. But if that isn't possible, here are some simple ones to start on.

YOGA EXERCISES

*The Corpse:* This is the most basic posture, and the one with which you should end every yoga session. Although it looks easy, you must concentrate to achieve the effect of calmness. Just lie on the floor, on a thick blanket if possible, making sure you are warm and comfortable. Draw your toes up towards you: towards your torso, stretching the heels, then relax your feet so that they flop out sideways. Rest your arms slightly away from your body, with the palms facing upward (if this is not comfortable, put your hands however suits you best). If necessary place a small cushion or pillow under your head or under the small of your back. Make sure your body is straight and symmetrical between the left and right sides. Now consciously relax each group of muscles up your body and remain like this for about five minutes. If you notice any distracting sounds, just say to yourself, "These sounds do not matter." (See illustration.)

*The Thunderbolt:* This is another simple posture. Sit back on your heels, hands resting on your knees, eyes looking straight ahead, with your head feeling as if it is being pulled up by a thread attached to the crown. If sitting on your heels is not very comfortable, try using a cushion or pillow to raise your buttocks slightly off the floor and to relieve tension in your knees and ankles. Or use a meditation stool if you have one. Focus your gaze on an object ahead of you and breathe evenly in and out for a few minutes. (See illustration.)

When you feel quite calm and peaceful, try

***The Lion:*** Remaining in the same position as for The Thunderbolt, open your eyes and mouth as wide as possible, stick your tongue out towards your chin, and give a loud ROAR! Doing this two or three times can bring a wonderful sense of relieving tension.

***The Tree:*** This is another very relaxing posture and much easier than it looks. There are several variations, and two are illustrated here. The sense of balance will probably come quickly, but to begin with you might feel more stable if you lean your back against a wall. It is easier to hold the position if your feet and legs are bare. Bend your right knee. Taking your right foot in both hands, place it against the inside of your left knee or higher if you can manage it. Press the sole of the right foot well into the left leg. Now, looking straight ahead, raise your hands above your head and place the palms together above your head. Hold this for as long as you feel comfortable, then repeat with the left foot against the right leg, and all the time looking straight ahead as far away as possible.

A variation is to raise the left leg behind you, holding it with your left hand, while raising your right arm. Then repeat the posture, holding your right leg behind you and raising your left arm. Again, look straight ahead all the time. (See illustrations.)

***The Triangle:*** Face forward, legs wide apart, arms out sideways level with your shoulders. Turn your right foot out and your left foot in. Now bend to the right, sliding your right hand down your right leg until it reaches as far as it comfortably will; this may be flat on the floor, or grasping your ankle, or placed against your knee. At this stage, only reach as far as you can easily. Without turning your hips, look up at your left hand, which should be raised vertically above you. Hold for as long as you can, then repeat, reversing the instructions to the left. (See illustration.)

***Salute to the Sun:*** This is an ancient Chinese exercise, traditionally done first thing in the morning to tone up the muscles and make you feel good for the day. It combines six yoga postures in a sequence of ten movements, and four of the positions are repeat-

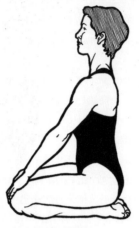

**THUNDERBOLT**
looking straight ahead

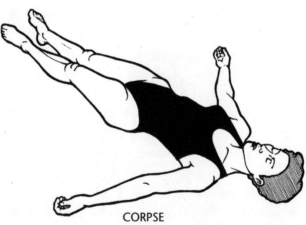

**CORPSE**
eyes closed and fingers relaxed

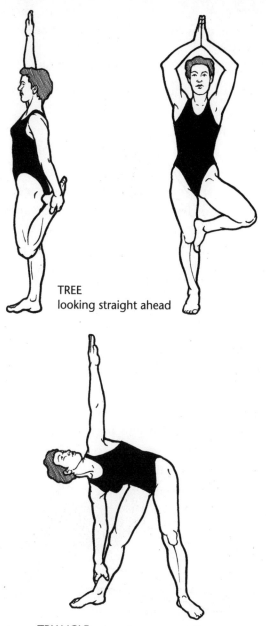

TREE
looking straight ahead

TRIANGLE
looking at raised left hand and with
hand grasping ankle, or lower leg

ed. You might find it easier to remember the sequence if you record the instructions in a soothing voice, allowing short pauses between each movement.

To begin with, you might find it easier if you ignore the breathing instructions and then include them when you feel more familiar with the routine.

1. Stand with your feet together, knees straight, back stretched up but not tense. Place the palms of your hands together in front of your chest and breathe in slowly and deeply. Breathe out as you move into the second position.

2. Bend forward from the hips until your hands are on the ground a short distance in front of you. Move your hands forward until your legs are straight. Tuck in your chin towards your chest and pull your stomach in. Then breathe in as you move into the third position.

3. Keeping your hands and arms in the same place, stretch one foot as far as you can behind you. At the same time, bend your other knee and bringing it forward between your arms, lifting up your head and slightly arching your back. Breathe out as you move to the fourth position.

4. Take your other foot back level with the first and straighten both legs. Try to press your heels toward the ground. Drop your head down so that your chin is tucked into your chest. Keep your arms straight and try to flatten and extend your spine. Take another breath in and breathe out as you go into the fifth position.

5. Keeping your hands and feet where they are, bend your arms and lower your body to the ground, touching the ground with your toes, knees, chest, and forehead. Pull your stomach in as you breathe out.

6. As you breathe in, lift up your head and bend backward, straightening your arms and legs so that the weight of your whole body is on your hands and toes.

7. As you breathe out, lift your bottom into the air, drop your head, tuck your chin in toward your chest, and straighten your legs. (This is the same as position four.)

8. As you breathe in, bring one leg forward so that the foot rests as closely as possible between your hands. Look up and bend back as in position three. Breathe out fully as you move into position nine.

9. Bring the other foot forward next to the first. Straighten your legs and tuck your chin in. (This is a repeat of position two.)

10. Breathe in as you lift your hands off the ground and stand up with a straight back. Join the palms in front of your chest.

You can repeat the sequence as many times as you like, though it is best to start gradually. (This variation of Salute to the Sun is taken from *Yoga* by Sophy Hoare.)

# 5

# *Alternative Medicine and IBS*

## Alternative Medicine: How It Can Help Your Irritable Bowel

> Surely here must be a golden opportunity for practitioners of
> alternative medicine and devotees of the holistic approach. The
> traditionalists have not much to boast about.
> —Letter in *The Lancet*, 1985

When you consider the statistics, it's evident that alternative medicine is, in fact, the first choice for Americans more often than conventional medicine is. According to the *Journal of the American
Medical Association* (11/11/98), at some point in the 1990s the total
number of visits to alternative practitioners surpassed the number
of visits Americans made to primary care physicians—by 1997, we
visited alternative practitioners nearly twice as often. More women
than men seek these therapies, but overall, four out of ten people
in the United States use some form of alternative medicine, spending billions of dollars in the process.

Most people who use alternative medicine are seeking remedies for chronic conditions. Homeopathy, herbal medicine, hypnotherapy, Chinese medicine and acupuncture, naturopathy,
ayurvedic medicine and most of the other alternative practices can

be effective for dealing with a wide range of problems, including Irritable Bowel Syndrome, because they emphasize treatment of the whole person rather than simply suppressing symptoms. They tend to be comprehensive in their approach, looking at all of the factors that contribute to the patient's health or illness over a period of time, which makes them especially effective at treating a chronic syndrome such as IBS. This doesn't mean the same system will work for everyone, but with patience and a willingness to explore the options, good results are likely.

Let us now look at how different forms of alternative medicine can help IBS. If you have had it for some time, it is unlikely that over-the-counter alternative remedies will have complete long-term success. Your condition is probably quite deep-seated; to heal it will most likely involve discussion about many aspects of your life with a therapist trained to discover the underlying cause. So you would be well advised to arrange for a personal consultation with a trained practitioner.

How do you know which form of alternative medicine to try? Unfortunately, there is no way of knowing which will work best for you. There are many paths to the same goal. Any therapy (whether conventional or alternative) has a placebo effect—that is, it may work just because you hope it will. But with something as long-term as IBS, in the end you will have to discover whatever is right for you.

You can start by asking friends—especially friends with IBS—whether they have had any success with alternative therapies. If your doctor is sympathetic to alternative medicine, she may recommend someone, although many doctors will only feel comfortable recommending alternative practitioners who are also MDs. Choose a therapist either because you have heard well of him or her or because the form of treatment appeals to you in some way. And keep an open mind about the different approaches.

It is not necessary to know about the philosophy behind any particular branch of alternative medicine for it to work. Nor is it necessary for you to have a firm belief that it will work. After all, many practitioners successfully treat children and even animals although these patients can have no expectation of what will happen. You should, however, feel open to allowing it to work and to being an active agent in your own recovery. It would be rather self-defeating to say, "I am using acupuncture to make me well, so therefore I don't need to do anything for myself." A more positive and probably more successful approach would be to say, "By seeing an acupuncturist I am taking a positive step toward helping myself."

The forms of alternative medicine that are known to have a good degree of success with IBS are homeopathy, medical herbalism, osteopathy, hypnotherapy, and acupuncture.

## Homeopathy

*Homeopathy* means "treat like with like." This means that a substance that in concentrated form brings out a certain reaction (say, a high fever) in a healthy person will, in a greatly diluted form, cure the same or similar symptoms in an unhealthy person. In this respect it is similar to vaccination. Introduce a diluted form of, say, diphtheria into the body, and this will enable the body to fight that disease.

Whereas conventional medicine suppresses symptoms, homeopathy regards symptoms as part of the body's attempt to fight disease; therefore symptoms must be respected and not suppressed.

Like most forms of alternative medicine, homeopathy is safe and does not produce side effects. The results tend to be long-lasting. You may notice an improvement quite quickly, or it may take longer. As a general guide, reckon that improvement will take about one month for each year that you have had the condition; so if you have had IBS for four years, it may take about four months to see a great improvement. If there are also deep-seated psychological or other problems, it could take even longer. The homeopath will probably warn you that your symptoms may get worse before they get better. Surprisingly, this is a good sign—it shows that the remedy is working. If your symptoms get significantly worse, you may be advised to stop taking the remedy just until the symptoms subside. But be assured that if you follow all the guidance the homeopath gives you, the results should be long-lasting.

You will be surprised at the questions the homeopath asks you: What sort of weather do you like or dislike? Do you prefer rivers or mountains? Do you prefer company or solitude? Warm or cold rooms? To get exercise or not? Do you like foods that are sweet or savory or salty or fatty? What skin problems have you had? Do you express emotions? What were your parents like? All these give an indication of the sort of person you are. The homeopath will want to know details of your past medical history, previous operations, general health, and recurring problems.

After taking all these into account, he will give you a remedy that is right for your particular constitution and personality. He may or may not give you something specifically for your irritable bowel. If he doesn't, that doesn't matter at all. The homeopath is trying to remove the underlying disturbance that causes the symptoms rather than treat the symptoms directly. What matters is the whole you.

Homeopathic tablets need to be taken rather differently from ordinary tablets. Do not handle them—just tip two tablets into the lid of the container and pop them straight into your mouth without touching them. Suck or chew them—do not swallow them whole. Make sure you do not eat or drink anything for twenty to thirty minutes before and after taking the tablets. While taking a course of homeopathic tablets, avoid all strong flavors, such as coffee, alcohol, cough sweets, mints, and strong toothpaste. Store the tablets away from all strong flavors and smells.

After taking a course of homeopathic medicine, you will usually feel very much better in yourself. You will almost certainly experience a greatly increased sense of well-being, and whether or not your irritable bowel improves rapidly, you will probably feel better able to cope with it. This is a typical response to homeopathic treatment.

Although IBS will almost certainly require specialist treatment to achieve success, in mild cases that have started quite recently it might be worth trying the following homeopathic remedies (which are available from many pharmacies and health food stores):

## COLICKY STOMACH PAIN

*Argentum nitricum:* for pain that gets worse when anticipating any kind of ordeal

*Colocynthis:* for pain that you can't keep still with and is eased by firm pressure or by doubling over

*Dioscorea:* for pain eased by stretching backwards or forwards

*Ipecacuanha:* for "cutting" pain and a feeling of nausea with each spasm

*Magnesia phosphorica:* for sharp, cramping pains that are relieved by warmth

*Mercurius solubilis:* for heavy mucus

## CONSTIPATION

Consider these remedies in addition to changes in your diet, more exercise, and a routine that encourages regularity:

*Aesculus or Nux vomica:* when there is a feeling of fullness even after a bowel movement

*Opium* (homeopathic opium, not the sort that is smoked in opium dens!): where overuse of laxatives has caused the bowel muscle to become ineffective

*Silica:* for stools that are hard to pass

## DIARRHEA

*Colocynthis:* for colicky pain that causes you to double over

*Natrum sulphuricum:* for morning diarrhea, loose and urgent

*Petroleum* (the homeopathic sort, not the kind in cars!): for diarrhea that worsens after cabbage and green vegetables

## DISTENSION OF ABDOMEN

*Carbo vegetabilis:* for gas that is difficult to bring up

*Cinchona officinalis:* if belching does not make it better

*Lycopodium:* for stomach pain and a feeling of fullness after only a little food

*Magnesia phosphorica:* for distension with cramping stomach pain

*Pulsatilla:* for gas, nausea, and the need to loosen clothing

*Sulfur:* for offensive-smelling gas

## STOMACH PAIN, LIKE INDIGESTION

*Dioscerea:* for colicky pain that gets better by straightening up or bending backwards

*Muriatic acid:* if pain is caused by taking indigestion tablets

*Nux vomica:* if pain is caused by nervous strain and usually occurs about two hours after eating

*Pulsatilla* or *Calcium carbonica:* especially after eating fatty or oily food

*Sulfur:* if you regurgitate your food, often about one hour after meals

These remedies cover simply the outward symptoms of IBS and take no account of aspects of your personality and lifestyle that may have contributed to it. Only a qualified homeopath can decide which "constitutional" remedy is right for your personality.

It is not easy to recommend which potency of tablets should be taken, or how often. So if you have never taken a homeopathic remedy before, you'd be better off consulting a qualified homeopath rather than buying a remedy over the counter.

# Herbal Medicine

The medical herbalist will help you to restore health and reintroduce a sense of internal balance. She will also encourage you to develop a lifestyle that will help you adapt more successfully to life's stresses and strains.

The main healing tool for the medical herbalist is, as you might have guessed, medicinal herbs. Many of today's conventional drugs have their basis in herbal medicine, but because of the way they are manufactured and processed, many of the original beneficial qualities of the herbs are lost.

Plant medicines are most commonly prescribed in liquid form as tinctures, fluid extracts, or syrups but may sometimes be given dried or as infusions, decoctions, tablets, or capsules. They may also be prescribed as ointments, lotions, and poultices. Used correctly, they do not bring on damaging side effects.

As with conventional medicine, you will first need to exclude any possibility of such conditions as diverticular disease, cancer, ulcerative colitis, or Crohn's disease. You should also identify any food allergies or intolerance to dairy products.

The aim of the medical herbalist will be to relax the central nervous system so that normal movement of the colon can be achieved without excessive spasm. This will be done with the use of plants that have antispasmodic, relaxing, or sedative qualities. Examples of plants that may be chosen are

—Anise seed (*Pimpinella anisum*)

—Bayberry (*Myrica cerifera*)

—Betony (*Stachys betonica*)

—Chamomile (*Matricaria recutita*)

—Comfrey (*Symphytum officinale*)

—Lavender (*Lavendula officinalis*)

—Peppermint (*Mentha piperata*)

—Valerian (*Valeriana officinalis*)

—Wild thyme (*Thymus serpyllum*)

—Wild yam (*Dioscorea villosa*)

A bulking agent such as psyllium seeds may be helpful, especially in the diarrhea form of IBS, to produce a normal bowel movement. The use of demulcent mucilaginous plants such as marshmallow root (*Althaea radix*) may also be prescribed.

Peppermint oil capsules provide effective relief for significant numbers of IBS sufferers, as a 1997 research study demonstrated. In this study, 79 percent of the IBS patients who took peppermint oil capsules experienced a reduction in the severity of their abdominal pain, with 29 percent becoming completely free of pain. Most of the patients (83 percent) had reduced bowel movements, less abdominal gurgling (73 percent of the patients) and less gas (79 percent of the patients).

In contrast with conventional medical practice, you may be advised not to take rough high-residue foods such as nuts and high-fiber cereals and to try instead root vegetables such as carrots, potatoes, rutabagas, parsnips, turnips, or various Caribbean or African vegetables.

When you work with a qualified herbalist, as with most forms of alternative medicine, you will be treated as a complete person: mind, body, and spirit. You will not be regarded as just a collection of digestive symptoms. No two people are the same, so you will receive an individual prescription based on your case history and the most appropriate path to health for you.

Some herbs can be harmful, especially during pregnancy, so make sure the practitioner you consult is properly qualified. **Self-help is not recommended.**

## Naturopathy

Naturopathic medicine is a comprehensive system that draws from a wide range of sources, including homeopathy, herbal medicine, acupuncture and nutritional therapy. Following principles of the healing power of nature, the importance of treating the whole person and of causing no harm, naturopathic doctors aim to treat underlying causes of illness rather than suppress symptoms. They consider education a major component of their approach and work with patients to promote good health and prevent illness.

Naturopathic practitioners are licensed after rigorous training that includes Western medical studies. A licensed N.D. will be fully acquainted with conventional medical techniques and should be able to offer sophisticated diagnostic methods. Treatment will be specifically tailored to your needs, always employing the least invasive means available. Since the aim is to treat the whole person, psychology and counseling are also important elements of naturopathic medicine.

Generally, a naturopath will begin treatment by interviewing the patient extensively, perhaps asking questions that seem beyond the scope of a specific condition such as IBS. This is to get a thorough sense of the patient's temperament and emotional disposition as well as medical history, since these factors inform the naturopath's design of a treatment.

With IBS, a naturopath will typically test you for specific food intolerances and help you plan a special diet and stress-reduction program, modifying these in further sessions according to the progress of your healing. You may be given a prescription for herbal medication and supplements (psyllium, peppermint oil, fennel seeds, slippery elm bark, skullcap, evening primrose oil or wormwood, for example) or for homeopathic remedies. Naturopaths also have training in acupuncture and Eastern medicine, and may incorporate these approaches in a treatment regimen.

## Osteopathy

Like other holistic approaches to disease, osteopathy tries to find out why the patient has a particular problem at a particular time. It is the reasons behind the disease that influence the osteopath and the way he will treat the patient.

One of the main tenets of osteopathy was laid down in 1870 by Andrew Taylor Still, the founding father of osteopathy. He maintained that structure governs function. In other words, if a thing is built correctly and is correctly adjusted and maintained, it will do the job it is supposed to do. If, however, it is treated badly and not looked after, then it will break down and fail.

Osteopaths believe that the bones and muscles of the body, and its surrounding nerves and blood vessels, are more than just the framework that supports the organs. They believe that the bones and muscles facilitate good health by a system of reflexes and muscle chains that allow the organs to be suspended correctly within the abdomen, the pelvis, and the chest cavity. When this supporting system is overloaded or abused, it will fail, and the organs connected to it will not work properly. If this continues for too long, abnormalities and disease can occur.

Take, for example, the gut, and especially the large intestine. The function of the large intestine is to collect solid waste matter and to store it while water is reabsorbed and minerals are recovered. The passage of this waste matter down the gut is a carefully controlled series of steps allowing digestion to take place in an orderly fashion. To facilitate communication between the digestive system and the brain, a series of nerve pathways send messages back and forth between the digestive organs and the spinal tissues.

The osteopath, using her knowledge of anatomy and physiology, together with her skill at feeling the tissues and muscles in the spine and abdomen, can diagnose and detect when things are not as they should be. She manipulates the nerve pathways in an attempt to change or influence anything that is not working properly in the gut. Because IBS is a disorder in which abnormal reflexes, often caused by stress, lead to the malfunctioning of the bowel, the osteopath attempts to treat the condition by using the reflexes themselves.

She also looks at the muscular "box" that encloses the abdominal organs. The "box" consists of the pelvic floor below, the diaphragm above, and the abdominal muscles all around. In normal breathing, the diaphragm massages the gut from above, and the downward force exerted by the diaphragm is received by the muscles of the pelvic floor. If these muscles are too tight or too loose, perhaps because of stress or childbirth, then this "massaging" action does not take place efficiently. Therefore, when treating cases of IBS, the osteopath will want to examine and treat the diaphragm and pelvic floor.

Like other holistic practitioners, the osteopath will emphasize the importance of a suitable diet, especially the inclusion of plenty of fiber, and the development of unhurried toilet habits.

Osteopathy definitely does not lend itself to self-help, and you should be sure that the osteopath you visit is adequately qualified. An inexperienced or unqualified person could do a lot of harm. Look for the qualification D.O. (Doctor of Osteopathy).

## Hypnotherapy

Hypnotherapy is a form of psychotherapy that uses hypnosis as an aid. It is a far cry from the stage performer who hypnotizes members of the audience for entertainment and amusement. Controlled studies have shown improvement in the symptoms of IBS from hypnotherapy.

Hypnotherapy cannot be forced on someone against his will, and the hypnotist has no power over his patient. He cannot extract from you things that you wish to keep secret nor make you do anything that you do not want to do. Under hypnosis you do not become unconscious nor do you fall asleep.

Hypnosis simply induces a very pleasant state of relaxation, which is particularly beneficial where symptoms have been induced or aggravated by stress. Most people are surprised at how relaxing and pleasant the sensation is. The hypnotist will enable you to draw on inner resources and be open to suggestions that encourage a new way of looking at life's problems.

He will endeavor to get at the cause of the problem and help you to resolve it. He does not treat symptoms directly. In the case of IBS, the cause will usually be some form of stress. He will regard your IBS as due to some disharmony within you and will work with you to rediscover harmony. He may also spend time suggesting ways in which you can control the intestinal smooth muscle, which is going into spasm and causing you pain.

Perhaps he will ask you to place your hand on your abdomen, to imagine that this hand is holding a warm hot water bottle, and to learn to relate this sensation of warmth to gaining control over your gut.

To cope with the pain of IBS, the hypnotherapist may ask you to form in your mind an image of the pain in whatever way comes most naturally to you. It may be in the form of an animal or a color or a shape; everyone's image is different. Then he may ask you to notice the first change that happens as the pain begins to diminish by one-tenth. This technique can be extremely helpful in reducing pain.

The hypnotherapist may show you how to enter and use an altered state of consciousness called *self-hypnosis*. He may give you appropriate autosuggestions to enable you to slow down or speed up the workings of your bowel. The relaxation induced in hypnosis allows your unconscious mind to receive and use suggestions that will be acceptable to you. After learning this technique, you will be able to do it on your own whenever you feel you need it. It may help you become more and more in control of your bowel. It is important that the suggestions and techniques of hypnosis and self-hypnosis be taught to you by a trained hypnotherapist.

Many people with IBS find hypnotherapy extremely beneficial, particularly for stomach pain and distension, and say it increases their feelings of general well-being. Some therapists see patients individually; others use group therapy. Recent research shows both these methods to be equally effective.

There are no medically recognized qualifications in hypnotherapy, and anyone can call himself a hypnotherapist. Medically qualified therapists are not necessarily better, but many people feel more confident if they know the person they see is also a professional doctor.

## Chinese Medicine and Acupuncture

According to traditional Chinese medicine, the symptoms of IBS make up a simple and typical syndrome, which has been treated effectively with Chinese herbs and acupuncture for thousands of years. Practitioners of Chinese medicine are trained in use of both herbs and acupuncture, and may use either or both in treatment, according to the particular needs of the patient. There is evidence that acupuncture can alter the contraction within the bowel.

Chinese medicine works with principles of life-energy, circulation and balance, describing physical conditions in terms of heat and cold, wet and dry, and other pairs of opposites that correspond to the universal yin and yang. The Chinese tradition describes yin as the receptive, cool, dark, moist, feminine force and yang as the active, warm, bright, dry, masculine force. The terms "feminine" and "masculine" here don't mean that women are all yin and men are all yang—in fact, the basis of health for everyone, according to Chinese medicine, is keeping yin and yang balanced and flowing within each bodily system and in each "organ." ("Organ" is in quotation marks here because in Chinese medicine the word describes a function, not a specific body part. So "kidney" refers to a particular set of cleansing and purifying functions, not to the mass of cells that form what Westerners call a kidney.)

Circulation plays a crucial role in Chinese medicine—not just circulation of blood, but of chi, life-energy. Blockages in the flow of chi, along with imbalances, account for most physical ailments. The goal of the acupuncturist is to restore and maintain balance and good circulation of the vital energy. When this goal is achieved, good health results.

The syndrome in Chinese medicine that corresponds to IBS results from a deficient or sluggish "spleen," with associated problems in the "stomach," "liver" and "kidneys." The "spleen" is responsible for key digestive functions. A deficient "spleen" can't metabolize food efficiently, which creates a "damp" condition in the body. The practitioner addresses the problem by using herbs and acupuncture to strengthen the spleen function, making it more efficient so it can clear and clean the entire digestive tract and "dry" the "dampness" within the body. The specific needs of the patient, including secondary symptoms and any relevant dietary or lifestyle factors, will determine the details of treatment.

Your first consultation with a Chinese medical practitioner is likely to last an hour or more. The diagnostic procedures may include a highly specialized pulse-reading, in which the acupuncturist checks 12 separate pulses in your wrist. This is a subtle and accurate diagnostic tool: a trained practitioner can discern strengths and weaknesses, blockages and imbalances in all parts of the body by "listening" to your pulse. Additionally, you may be asked for a urine sample, and you will probably be encouraged to talk about what you believe initially triggered your IBS, and to look at what might be causing you anger or anxiety. Chinese medicine has always recognized that emotions can be a factor in physical disease, though this concept has only recently been accepted in Western medicine. Like so much alternative medicine, acupuncture works on the basis of treating the cause and allowing the cure to occur by itself. The effects of acupuncture are therefore long-lasting, provided you take reasonable care of yourself.

The practitioner may recommend changing to a different diet, adapted to your particular disharmony—avoiding or reducing coffee, refined foods, cheese and dairy products, alcohol, spicy foods, and meat. If you have gas, you may have to eliminate cabbage, legumes, peas, beans, and Brussels sprouts. Since so many people with IBS tend to be in a hurry or to eat inadequate meals, you will be encouraged to eat a wholesome, nutritious diet with plenty of greens (such as spinach), rice cakes instead of bread, and fluids taken half an hour before and after food rather than during a meal.

You may be asked to keep a record of what you eat during the week, together with details of the symptoms particular foods may produce. Once you have discovered what disagrees with you, you will be encouraged to introduce different foods gradually.

You may be prescribed a regimen of herbs, acupuncture sessions or both. For the acupuncture treatment, the practitioner will choose about three or four acupuncture points that directly harmonize the colon. Most likely these will be on the forearm, feet, legs, abdomen or lower back. She will insert very thin needles, about the thickness of a hair, a few millimeters deep into those points. The needles are left in place for about fifteen minutes. When they are inserted by a skilled practitioner, you will hardly be aware of them. Unused sterile needles are used for each patient, and there should be no bleeding or swelling, since the acupuncture points are not situated over blood vessels or vital organs. It does not hurt, unless you are so tense that you aggravate it. So once again, your state of mind influences your healing.

You will probably need about three sessions of treatment, together perhaps with a course of Chinese herbal medicine. After that, some people feel a need to return about three times a year to keep their ailment under control. As with homeopathy, it may take about one month for each year you have had IBS to get a real improvement, so persevere.

As with other forms of alternative medicine, acupuncture will affect the way you feel as a whole person and will aim to enhance your overall state of health. In ancient China, doctors were paid to keep their patients healthy rather than to treat them when they were sick, and acupuncture was one of the traditional methods of maintaining a state of health.

## Other Forms of Alternative Medicine

Homeopathy, herbal medicine, osteopathy, hypnotherapy, and acupuncture are the main forms of alternative medicine for which I know practitioners are optimistic that they can treat IBS with some hope of success. There are, however, many other forms of holistic medicine that are suitable for digestive problems in general.

## SHIATSU

Shiatsu is a form of massage based on principles of Chinese medicine. As in acupuncture, the key to health is balance, which occurs when the body's vital energy flows freely. Practitioners follow a map of the body that traces meridians, or energy pathways, throughout the body. A shiatsu massage may help relieve immediate pain, but its primary intent is to unblock the meridians and let the vital energy flow. This leads to overall physical well-being and helps provide a sense of emotional stability and balance.

A shiatsu practitioner may focus on a particular region of the body or may determine that a full-body treatment is more appropriate. In either situation, shiatsu can improve circulation and digestion and is an effective way to reduce stress.

## REFLEXOLOGY

Reflexology works by applying pressure and massage to the feet. Practitioners work with the premise that there are clearly defined points on the feet that form lines of energy linking with every part of the body. When these pressure points are manipulated, there will be an improvement in the organ to which the pressure point is linked.

A skilled practitioner can tell by massaging the different areas of your feet where in the rest of your body you have problems, because you will feel some discomfort in the area of your foot that relates to the ailing area of your body.

Although you will probably get most benefit by visiting a practitioner of reflexology, it is possible to do a certain amount yourself or to have someone do it for you.

The success of reflexology may work on the same principle as acupuncture—that is, pressure at the end of a line of energy may release chemicals called *endomorphins*, which reduce pain and can induce a feeling of well-being. It is also possible that by stimulating the nerve endings, the functioning of different organs will benefit.

The sole of the right foot has an area that corresponds to the ascending colon, and the sole of the left foot an area that corresponds to the descending colon. (See illustration.) The transverse colon that goes across the center of your abdomen is shared between each foot. If these parts of the feet are carefully massaged in the same direction in which food travels through the colon, this may cause the whole colon area to improve greatly.

If you would like to try it for yourself, this is what you do. Find a sitting position in which you can comfortably massage the soles of your feet.

One possible way is sitting on a chair in such a way that you can place each foot in turn on the thigh of the other leg. Starting with your right foot, place it comfortably on our left thigh (or in any other position that allows easy massage). Place your left thumb in the area shown on the drawing and massage gently with your thumb up the foot and then across to the edge in the direction of the arrows. As you do this, visualize the corresponding area in your abdomen—up the right side and across the middle. Do this gently several times, always working in the same direction. Then massage the area representing the sigmoid colon, working from the outside of the foot to the inside as in the drawing.

RIGHT FOOT                    LEFT FOOT

Ascending colon — Transverse colon — Descending colon

Start with thumb here — Sigmoid flexure

Now place your left foot comfortably on your right thigh (or wherever else is easiest for you). Bearing in mind that you are attempting to follow the natural direction of the digested food in the colon, place your right thumb on the instep area of the foot, then across to the outside, and down toward the heel in the direction shown on the drawing. Do this gently several times, always working in the same direction. As before, visualize your own colon, from the center of your abdomen and down the left side toward the rectum. Then massage the area representing the sigmoid colon, working from the outside of the foot to the inside.

Finally gently massage the underside of all your toes, working from the top of each toe to the ball of the foot.

As you work on the colon area of your foot, you may feel discomfort, perhaps a prickly feeling or the sensation of grains of sand under the skin. This is an indication that the area of your colon (bowel) is in need of attention; by working gently as described, you may notice a considerable improvement in your digestion.

Find time to do these exercises each morning and evening, for five to ten minutes. Take care not to apply too much pressure— this might increase tension in your colon.

## AUTOGENIC TRAINING

This is an extension of hypnotherapy, but at a self-help level. You can put ideas into your own mind that can help your own healing. Many people feel upset, even insulted, when their doctor tells them their irritable bowel is caused by a state of mind. The label "psychosomatic illness" conjures up all the wrong images. This is where autogenic training can be particularly useful.

Most doctors will accept that a state of mind can cause a physical illness, and a persistent physical illness can produce an upset state of mind. Now if your mind can affect your body in a harmful way (as with IBS), can you make the mental leap that your mind can also affect your body in a beneficial way? If a poor state of mind can cause IBS, perhaps a good state of mind can improve it. There is proven scientific evidence to show that autogenics can help to reduce high blood pressure and increase mental well-being.

Autogenic training uses the mind to help the body. A sort of "mind-over-matter" cross between self-hypnosis and meditation, it really needs expert guidance, and you cannot easily learn it from books.

This simple introduction to self-hypnosis may be helpful to you. Relax, following one of the relaxation exercises in the "Exercises for Relaxation" section of this chapter. Then form a mental picture of anything pleasurable that occurs to you. Hold this in your mind, then let that image change into an image of yourself. Spend time building that image of yourself into someone who has the qualities you desire, such as tranquillity, freedom from stress, freedom from IBS. Then recall a time of your life when you were like this (possibly many years ago, even in childhood), and hold that image. Now project that image of yourself at that time into an image of yourself today and hold it. You were like that once, you can be like that again. Finally, visualize the "new" you doing the things you do now and coping well, without Irritable Bowel Syndrome.

Another method is to use an affirmation. Say to yourself, "I have control over my body," and then if you feel this isn't really true, say to yourself, "I haven't, because . . . ." Then say again, "I have control over my body," and again, "I haven't because . . . ." Continue until you have no further reasons to give. Then say to yourself, "My bowel is quiet and calm, and I can control it." As you say this, try hard to believe it. Place your hands on the area of your ascending and descending colon and generate a sense of warmth, quietness, and freedom from spasm.

Since self-healing involves a commitment to believing you can be well again, try these visualization exercises:

—Just try to see yourself well again. Visualize your IBS being overcome, in any way that makes sense to you.

—Focus on the smooth muscle that propels the digested food and is the cause of much of the trouble as it goes into spasm. Think about this area of muscle, visualize it moving in beautiful waves, with warmth, without spasm. Think of the sea, with a sailboat moving peacefully and gently along on the waves. Transfer this image to the smooth, wavelike motion of the muscles of your colon.

—Create in your mind an image of your bowel, in a way that you understand. It doesn't need to be medically accurate, just your own image of your insides. See your colon as a tube of smooth muscle going into painful spasm, the food in it getting held up, forming into pellets, and causing you pain. Then visualize the spasm disappearing, the food in the tube passing in gently rhythmic waves up the right side of your tummy across the middle and down the left side. See your body making itself well again. If you are on prescribed medicines (antispasmodics or bulk laxatives), see them working in your gut. Visualize the effect all this has, giving you normal stools, freedom from pain, freedom to eat whatever you want, relaxation. See the behavior of your irritable bowel as weak and your body's defenses as strong and under your control. Do this exercise two or three times a day. Believe in it. It really does work.

As with all forms of meditation, don't expect instant results. Practice these exercises regularly, and over time you will be surprised at the change in you.

## AYURVEDA

Ayurveda means "the science of life" and has been the basis of traditional medicine in India for thousands of years. Its chief concern is balance: the universe is seen as a combination of five elements (fire, earth, air, water and ether) that complement each other in a dynamic interplay. Human physiology is a combination of these elements, and all physical well-being depends on their harmonious interaction. Beyond simply addressing physical symptoms, Ayurveda considers emotional, mental and spiritual components inextricable from a person's health.

The key factor, according to Ayurveda, is digestion. This applies not only to food but also to how we assimilate, or digest, new experiences, trauma, excitement—in other words, how we deal with stress. According to Ayurveda, each person has a specific constitutional type, which determines how we digest and serves as the basis for diagnosing problems. Dietary changes, as well as herbal remedies and other treatments, are prescribed to rebalance the constitution.

In an examination the Ayurvedic practitioner will take a detailed medical history and will ask questions that help ascertain the particularities of your constitution. He or she will also probably examine your tongue, eyes and pulse in much more detail than a Western doctor would. You will likely be asked to produce a urine sample as well.

Ayurvedic treatment emphasizes balancing the patient's constitution as a whole rather than simply addressing specific symptoms. For IBS this will probably include dietary modification and may make use of medicinal herbs, fasting, sweating and special oil treatments.

## BIOFEEDBACK

Biofeedback works with the body's own mechanisms to relieve stress by monitoring the body with special machines. These instruments measure muscle movements, skin temperature, heart rate, sweat gland activity and brainwave activity. When a pattern of tension appears, the machine triggers a flashing light or beeper. The signals help you learn to take control of processes that are normally involuntary, by letting you observe areas that remain tense unnecessarily and then showing you when you've let go of the tension.

By working with biofeedback equipment, people can undo chronic patterns of stress, until they no longer need to rely on the monitors. IBS sufferers have found that biofeedback therapy can help relieve their symptoms and promote a general lessening of the condition—improvements that remain years after the therapy sessions.

## SOMATICS

In the past few decades, a number of innovators have developed profound healing techniques that demand we revise our concepts about the body and mind. These are therapies that often began as responses to physical injuries, but showed startling transformations in the psychological and emotional states of patients that prompted practitioners to investigate further. Among the techniques that have evolved from these investigations are the Feldenkrais Method, the Alexander Technique, Hakomi and Somatics, which have all shown good results in treating a wide range of conditions, both physical and psychological.

Building on the pioneering work of Hans Selye (who is credited with first identifying stress as a source of human illness) and Moshe Feldenkrais, Thomas Hanna developed a system of body-oriented therapy known as Somatics. Underlying Somatics is the observation that we continually respond to daily stresses and traumas—whether these are physical, emotional or of some other origin—with specific muscular reflexes. In other words, every time we experience fear, anxiety, anger, frustration, we contract specific muscles—often without awareness of our physical reaction.

When these muscular reflexes are triggered repeatedly, we have a harder time undoing the tension voluntarily, until the contractions become so habitual and ingrained that we forget how to release them. We become stuck, perhaps experiencing a great deal of pain. Hanna called this state of forgetfulness "sensory-motor amnesia," and considered it the basis of our chronic syndromes and functional disorders.

According to this view, everything that happens to us causes a necessary reaction in our central nervous system. Every muscular contraction has a nervous-system component. Our nervous systems and muscles lock into patterns that once helped us adapt to a difficult situation and are now very likely obsolete. Sensory-motor amnesia occurs when we become habituated to these obsolete patterns, holding onto tension that no longer serves any purpose.

In Somatics, the key to unlocking these debilitating patterns lies in a system of exercises that retrain our muscles and neurons to operate in ways we've become unaccustomed to. Some of the exercises move a region of the body or group of muscles further in the direction of the habitual clenching, in order to bring more conscious awareness to the region and re-establish voluntary control of the muscles. Other exercises retrain neural pathways by making unusual separations—for instance, moving head and eyes in different directions at once. All of the exercises are performed very gently and slowly, without straining.

Hanna was emphatic about treating the whole person rather than simply responding to specific ailments. Many of the Somatics exercises isolate specific muscle groups, but the exercises are meant to be done in sequences that integrate the entire body and mind. Similarly, though on the surface Somatics appears geared toward helping people with muscular conditions, a great many people have found it highly effective for healing chronic pain of all sorts, including psychological and emotional difficulties. This is probably because Somatics addresses the neural components of even our tiniest unconscious movements and helps us take control of aspects of our lives we had thought were beyond our participation.

The ramifications for treating IBS with Somatics are clear. At the very least, the system is an effective way of reducing stress without side effects. For some people, it may provide complete relief from ibs symptoms. Other benefits of the therapy include cessation of anxiety, improved energy, greater mental clarity and a general sense of well-being. Adherents of the exercises claim Somatics can actually reverse the aging process.

## BACH FLOWER REMEDIES

These remedies work by healing the negative states of mind that are thought to be the cause of physical disorders: anger, jealousy, fear, grief, hopelessness, terror, persistent unwanted thoughts, exhaustion, self-distrust, anxiety, irritability, depression, guilt, resentment, bitterness, intolerance, tension, and many others. Perhaps you can see some of your own feelings here—most people can. Your local health food store will probably carry Bach flower remedies or have information about how you can get them.

## AROMATHERAPY

Practitioners of aromatherapy administer essential oils to different parts of the body as a form of healing. These oils can help IBS in several ways, both as a direct treatment for the gut and as a means of controlling stress. The main method of use is general massage applied by a therapist, but you could learn from a qualified aroma-therapist how to apply the oil locally to the abdomen. You may also be given oils to put in your bath to promote relaxation. In addition, oils may be given as inhalants, tinctures, and lotions. They are never taken internally.

If you want to try it yourself, your local health food store and some pharmacies may have stocks of essential oils. It is important to use them correctly, since the wrong use may have the reverse effect or even provoke an unpleasant reaction. So seek good advice and follow it carefully. There are also several books available, which will guide you on which oils to use and how to use them.

# 6

## *You Are What You Eat*

## One Man's Wheat . . . A Look at Problem Foods

> There is now evidence to suggest that intolerance to specific foods—
> as distinct from allergy—is common and may be an important factor
> in the etiology [cause] of the Irritable Bowel Syndrome.
> —*Quarterly Journal of Medicine 52*, 1983

The foods that most commonly aggravate IBS are wheat and dairy (milk) products, although usually people find problems with one or the other rather than both. Of those whose IBS is caused by food intolerance, nearly half can trace it to one of these substances. (Coffee, corn, and onion come next, affecting 20 to 25 percent, with barley, chocolate, citrus fruits [oranges, lemons, limes, grapefruit], eggs, oats, potatoes, rye, tea, and yeast causing problems for 10 to 18 percent. A number of other foods affect less than 10 percent.)

Wheat and milk products are the most common foods eaten in Western countries. Most of us eat them every day and usually in every meal and snack in some form or other. It could just be the quantity and frequency of consumption that causes such widespread intolerance.

# Intolerance to Wheat

IBS-induced intolerance to wheat is not the same thing as celiac disease, which is a condition usually diagnosed in infancy and caused by the inability of the intestine to absorb the gluten in wheat, rye, barley, and oats. Celiac disease can be identified by medical testing, whereas IBS cannot. It's probably not the gluten in wheat that is the culprit for IBS, but research has yet to identify what is.

If wheat is only a minor problem to you, you may be all right if you eat it just once every few days. But if it causes serious IBS symptoms, you will have to avoid all wheat flour, refined or unrefined. Substitutes are cornmeal, millet flour, potato flour, rice flour, ground rice, rye flour, amaranth flour, quinoa flour or soy flour. You could also use buckwheat (no relation to wheat despite its name), millet, oatmeal, or whole oats. (See Appendix for a list of substitute foods.) Your local health food store will probably stock some of these. All the substitute flours cook differently from wheat flour, so experiment before you use them.

Because wheat is used in a wide variety of foods, you will need to read food labels carefully. If a product contains any of the following items, it could contain wheat:

| | |
|---|---|
| Cereal protein | Thickener |
| Corn flour | Thickening |
| Edible starch | Vegetable protein |
| Flour | Wheat meal |
| Modified starch | Wheat protein |
| Rusk | Whole grain flour |
| Starch | |

Many of the recipes in this book contain gluten-free flour. It is usually manufactured from rice, amaranth or quinoa, or else from wheat that has been processed to remove the gluten. Low-gluten spelt flour is another alternative that some people who have wheat allergies or intolerance can digest. Check with your local health food store.

Gluten-free cookbooks are available from libraries, book-stores, and health food stores, as are books written for people with celiac disease, which may contain recipes for substitute flours.

If you don't eat wheat or gluten for long periods of time, you may get a deficiency of B-group vitamins (thiamine, riboflavin, nicotinic acid, folic acid, pyridoxine, and vitamin B12). Ask your doctor about vitamin B supplements.

## Intolerance to Milk Products

Milk contains a naturally occurring sugar called lactose, which is broken down during digestion by an enzyme called lactase. Some people do not produce enough lactase, so they can't properly break down the lactose in milk products, and this can lead to pain and diarrhea. Patients with IBS are similarly affected by lack of lactase, which breaks down the lactose during digestion. However, more than 50 percent all humans lack this enzyme after puberty. Patients with IBS may have greater symptoms because of their visceral hypersensitivity.

Like wheat, dairy products (milk, butter, cheese, yogurt, and cream) are in many of the foods we eat, so check food labels carefully. As with wheat, dairy products come in various forms:

Calcium lactate

Casein

Lactic acid

Lactic acid esters

Sodium lactate

Whey

Whey solids

However, it is still perfectly possible to have a nutritious and fulfilling diet without these products. For example, goat's milk products will probably not upset you unless you have a serious allergy to all dairy products. Yogurts and most cheese have much less lactose than milk, and most people can take them, especially in small quantities. Heating milk to the boiling point can change some of the substances that trigger unpleasant symptoms, and evaporated milk is fine for many people, since its heat treatment destroys some of the proteins that cause problems.

If you really can't take any naturally occurring dairy products, soy milk is now widely available, and you will probably get used to it very quickly. It can be used as a substitute for milk in drinks, in cooking, and on cereal. Try to use soy milk that has been fortified with calcium. There are other lactose-free products on the market such as Lactaid and Dairy Ease.

Most soft margarines (including at least one brand of "soy margarine") contain whey, a milk byproduct. Substitutes that contain no dairy products are Spectrum Spread, Shedd's Willow Run Spread and Hain Pure Foods Soft Safflower Oil Margarine, kosher brands, and also tahini (ground sesame seeds) or some sunflower spreads. Some people find ghee (clarified butter) suits them. You can make it by melting some butter gently over low heat, allowing it to cool slightly, then pouring it carefully into another container, taking care to leave at the bottom of the saucepan the "scumlike" granules, which are the proteins that may cause problems to people who can't take dairy products. Keep it refrigerated. Ghee is also available in most Indian grocery stores.

If you eat little or no dairy products, you will need to replace milk's many important ingredients, especially calcium and vitamin A. Calcium is not easily available in other forms except supplement tablets, and is essential for the growth of bones and teeth and for important bodily processes such as blood clotting. It is especially important for girls and young women to take enough calcium to reduce the risk of osteoporosis in later years; yet these are the very years when they might cut down on dairy products if they perceive them as fattening. Soy milk contains no calcium (unless you buy a brand that is calcium fortified), so if in doubt, ask your doctor about calcium supplements. Teenagers should have 1200 mg of calcium a day, and women ages 20 to 40 should have 1000 mg a day. There are lactose-free milk products being sold today, such as Lactaid. Some of these are calcium enhanced and are viable alternatives.

## Intolerance to Other Foods

Irritable Bowel Syndrome is not the end of civilized eating as we know it. No matter what upsets your bowels, there are substitute foods available that are perfectly acceptable and that you will almost certainly get used to quickly (see Appendix).

If yeast is a problem, avoid alcoholic drinks, yeast spreads such as bread (except soda bread or any unleavened bread), yogurt, commercial fruit juices, all B-group vitamins (unless labeled "yeast-free"), and hydrolyzed vegetable protein.

To make shopping easier, write to the head office of your local supermarket and ask them which products they stock that do not contain the ingredients you cannot eat, especially if these are wheat or dairy products. They will be glad to send you a list of suitable alternatives.

## Food Allergy or Food Intolerance?

*Child:* Mom, what's a lergic?

*Mother:* A what?

*Child:* A lergic.

*Mother:* I don't know. Why?

*Child:* Because John in my class is allergic, and he doesn't have to eat school lunches.

Not having to eat school lunches may be an advantage to food allergies. Not being able to eat ordinary, everyday foods definitely isn't.

Do onions make your irritable bowel worse? How about oranges, cabbage, or coffee? Or perhaps milk, beer, breakfast cereals, or fried food? If so, take comfort—you are just like lots of other people who have IBS. After all, there is no doubt that some foods can make the condition worse for many people. Is this due to an allergy to those foods?

Perhaps when you have asked your doctor whether you might be allergic to the foods that are giving you problems, he or she has dismissed the idea and told you that your IBS is "all in your mind," and if only you worried less about it, your gut would return to normal.

It is certainly true that for most people their IBS becomes worse when they are under stress, and diet is a secondary factor. There are many sufferers whose symptoms are triggered more by their state of mind than by what they eat. A report on food additives presented to the British Royal College of Physicians in 1988 produced some interesting results and suggested that people may not be as sensitive to as many foods as they fear. During experiments, when people knew they were eating something that typically disagreed with them, they got unpleasant reactions. When they ate the same substances without knowing what they were eating, very few got unpleasant reactions. This, so far, is what other researchers have discovered. But the researchers in this experiment carried the tests further and concluded that if people eat something that they know will disagree with them, a certain level of anxiety is generated, which causes changes to take place in their body. These changes disrupt the digestive process and cause the intolerant reactions.

Perhaps the thought of having to eat out gets you worried. It is surprising how many people get IBS symptoms before they eat out, perhaps before they even leave the house. The symptoms are obviously not being caused by the food but simply by the worry of eating out.

This does not mean that, if you are one of these people, you are neurotic, obsessive, or overanxious. There is, indeed, a direct physical change taking place; it is not imaginary. But it is yet another example of how your state of mind is contributing directly to your irritable bowel.

There are four basic reactions to food:

1. You like it and eat it with no problems.

2. You have a *food aversion:* you dislike or avoid a particular food for purely psychological reasons (for example, you don't like to eat fat, meat, spicy foods, or "foreign" foods).

3. You have a *food allergy:* your immune system fights off certain substances in the food.

4. You have a *food intolerance:* the food causes unpleasant sensations in your system.

The next sections are concerned with the last two: food allergy and food intolerance.

## Food Allergy

An *allergy* is an adverse reaction involving the body's immune system. The body's response to whatever is causing the allergy is usually immediate and can be severe. The substance that causes the reaction is called the allergen.

Common allergens are

—Pollens and grasses

—House dust mites and their droppings

—Fur and feathers

—Foods and food additives

—Ingredients of clothing and cosmetics

—Certain drugs, such as penicillin

—Insect bites and stings

Typical conditions caused by allergy are asthma, some forms of eczema, hay fever, rhinitis (a constantly congested or runny nose), and urticaria (hives). It is interesting that many people with the diarrhea form of Irritable Bowel Syndrome also suffer from one or more of these typical allergic reactions. If you already have one of these conditions, it is likely that food allergy may be partially causing your abdominal symptoms; a diet that improves your IBS may well improve your allergy condition, too.

When you have an allergy, you develop antibodies to the allergens, and the antibodies react against the allergens by producing chemicals such as histamines, which cause typical allergic symptoms such as wheezing, a runny nose, or a rash. Doctors often prescribe antihistamines to overcome these unpleasant symptoms.

There are reliable tests to identify individual allergens, the two most common being the skinprick test and the RAST test.

## THE SKINPRICK TEST

This is the standard test for allergies. A small drop of the suspected allergen is placed on the arm, and a prick or scratch is made in the skin below the drop so that a small amount of the allergen enters the skin. If the patient is sensitive to the allergen, a noticeable reaction will appear on the skin. This test is not always conclusive.

## THE RAST (*RADIOALLERGOSORBENT*) TEST

This will usually follow a skinprick test. It measures the level of immunoglobulin E (IgE) antibodies that the patient has to a specific substance and thereby the extent to which he or she is allergic to it.

An individual's response to an allergen usually lasts for many years, perhaps even a lifetime, and can be caused even by tiny amounts of that allergen—in extreme cases by being in the same house with a cat or using a knife on which there is just a trace of butter.

Food allergy has the same reactions as any other sort of allergy. When you develop antibodies against a particular food, the food becomes the allergen, and the antibodies combine with that food to cause the unpleasant symptoms.

## Food Intolerance

Food intolerance is rather different. It is an adverse reaction to food, but the involvement of the immune system is unproven, because tests for allergy come back negative. This doesn't mean that immune reactions aren't involved, but it is unlikely that they are the main cause of the symptoms. So far, there is no single reliable test of food intolerance (but see pages 194–201 on the exclusion diet).

Some foods contain chemicals that upset some people, possibly by upsetting the balance of bacteria in the gut and by producing chemicals that cause the symptoms to develop. Conditions thought to be caused or aggravated by food intolerance are

—Constipation

—Crohn's disease

—Diarrhea

—Fatigue

—Hyperactivity in children

—Irritable Bowel Syndrome

—Joint pain

—Migraine

—Nausea

—Stomach and duodenal ulcers

—Vomiting

Culprit foods tend to be those that are consumed regularly (milk, wheat, coffee and onions, for example). This is one reason it can be difficult to identify the cause of IBS and why many people cannot trace the start of the symptoms to a particular time.

They usually just notice mild symptoms such as a headache, indigestion, or upset stomach that gradually get worse over a period of time. To make diagnosis even harder, symptoms may come and go, get better for a while, then get worse. Unlike food allergy, food intolerance may disappear if the offending food is avoided for several months and then taken only in small quantities (although it may recur if the food is then eaten frequently).

While it is true that intolerances can come and go, it is also true that avoiding one staple food may increase the use of another, and this increase in use can create a new sensitivity. The new food may not have bothered you when you ate it only occasionally, but by eating it in large quantities you may develop an intolerance to it. Be cautious, therefore, about eating new foods too frequently. You may also develop new intolerances that are triggered by antibiotics, viral infections, or gastroenteritis.

If you think your IBS is caused by allergy to any staple food like wheat or dairy products, ask your doctor if she can arrange an allergy test for you. If the test turns out to be negative, accept that you are not allergic to a food but that you may well have an intolerance to it.

## Which Foods Cause Which Reactions?

In order to discover which foods disagree with you, as a first step try this simple regime. For two weeks cut out completely all alcohol, coffee, fatty foods, fried foods, red meat, and no more than about two other things that you know for certain make your irritable bowel worse. In addition, have as few dairy products as you can. Just cutting out these things may make your IBS better enough to live with. Have a simple leisurely breakfast of fruit juice, cereal, and whole-grain toast with vegetable margarine and marmalade or honey. For lunch (or dinner) have whole-grain bread sandwiches, or salad, and fresh fruit. For dinner (or lunch) have a vegetarian meal, or fish, chicken, or lean meat with salad or fresh vegetables, followed by fresh fruit. Drink as little black tea and coffee as you can, and try to cut out alcohol and smoking. Use honey instead of sugar for sweetening.

Where irritable bowel is characterized by pain after meals, you may find it helpful to eat less fat and more protein, as fats can cause the muscles of the intestines to go into painful spasm.

If these suggestions make you feel better, try introducing other foods in small quantities at the rate of one every two days, noting any reactions these new foods provoke. With any luck, this slightly reduced diet should show you which foods are causing problems, and you can adjust your eating habits accordingly.

Some people feel they are so sensitive to so many foods that their lives become nothing but misery. They never eat out at friends' homes or in restaurants; they avoid events that include meals; they may even stop going on vacation; and they eat intolerably restricted diets. Their own lives, and their families' lives, become dominated by their irritable bowels.

Not eating what you like can be inconvenient, and having to avoid basic foods can lead to a disrupted lifestyle, a diminished social life, and even to undernutrition. So don't jump to instant conclusions about what does or doesn't agree with you. Although a few people find that many foods trigger their IBS symptoms, most find that they can manage quite well by avoiding just two or three. If you have any doubt about your diet, talk to your doctor or a dietician.

## Which Diet: High-Fiber or Low-Fiber?

The Irritable Bowel Syndrome is a common and poorly understood chronic condition that is treated with a great variety of drugs and other therapies without enduring success.

—*Gastroenterology* 95, 1988

You may be one of the lucky ones. You leave the doctor's office clutching a prescription for an antispasmodic, a bulk laxative (for constipation) plus, possibly, a short-term antidepressant (to reduce stress), and they may work well and greatly improve your IBS.

Or they may not. In the present state of medical knowledge, not only is there no single definitive test that your doctor can use and say, "This test is positive, therefore you have Irritable Bowel Syndrome," there is also no single therapy that is reliably effective in the general treatment of IBS. Until there is, you will have to make do with whatever conventional or alternative medicine can offer, or with the various things you can do to help yourself.

Unfortunately, there is also no one special diet to make the irritable bowel less irritable. Until quite recently, bran was the standard recommended effective treatment, but that is probably not as effective as was originally thought, and some people find it makes their condition worse. A high-fiber diet works well for a large proportion of IBS sufferers, while for a minority a low-fiber diet is better. Where a particular food is the cause of the problem, the diet will have to be specially modified.

## Our Current Dietary Habits

The typical American diet includes white bread, corn flakes, cakes, cookies, chocolate, pies, chips, frozen vegetables, canned fruit, black tea, coffee, and immense quantities of processed foods. Two hundred years ago, most of these foods were quite unknown to the general population, and so was IBS. Could there be a connection?

We eat about twice as many carbohydrates (including sugar) and half as much fiber as we need in our less active lives. We eat a lot more fat than is good for us, and we also consume an amazing cocktail of chemicals in processed food. Meat and other animal products may contain hormones and antibiotics. Is it surprising, then, that things start to go wrong inside our insides? In addition, most of us have been prescribed antibiotics at some time or other, sometimes quite frequently or for extended periods, and this may upset the balance of bacteria in the gut, killing off some useful bacteria and altering others so chemicals that aggravate IBS are produced. Candida, which can contribute to IBS symptoms, often flourishes under these conditions.

So what should you do? First, think carefully about your symptoms and follow the advice given in this book. Then consider how you can modify your diet. A high-fiber diet will usually help constipation; a low-fiber diet often helps diarrhea and gas; and specific problem foods can be identified with an exclusion diet.

## Constipation or Diarrhea?

Before deciding whether constipation or diarrhea is your main symptom, you should know exactly what these conditions are. Do you have several bowel movements every day? If so, is this really diarrhea? Or do you have one every few days, and if so, is this constipation?

True diarrhea is the passing of unformed watery stools, whether this happens frequently or not. True constipation is passing small hard stools and often involves straining at stool. Pseudodiarrhea may be described as having frequent bowel movements that are not unformed and watery, and may even be hard and pellety; pseudoconstipation might be having to strain to pass normally formed or even loose stools (types 5, 6, or 7 on the scale below). With pseudoconstipation you may also experience rectal dissatisfaction—the sensation after a bowel movement that there is more to come.

Dr. K. W. Heaton and his colleagues at Bristol Royal Infirmary in England have done some very interesting work on pseudodiarrhea and pseudoconstipation and have produced a simple method of helping their patients to decide which, if either, they have. They have devised the Bristol Stool Form Scale, and I am grateful to Dr. Heaton for permission to reproduce it here.

Over the next few days, look carefully at the stools you produce (at this point in reading this book, this should not embarrass you at all!) and see which description fits best.

The Bristol Stool Form Scale describes seven types of stool:

1. Separate, hard lumps like nuts

2. Sausage-shaped but lumpy stools

3. Stool like a sausage or snake but with cracks on its surface

4. Stool like a sausage or snake, smooth and soft

5. Soft, bloblike stool with clear-cut edges

6. Fluffy pieces with ragged edges; a mushy stool

7. Watery stool; no solid pieces

If descriptions 1, 2, and, to a much lesser extent, 3 describe your stools, this is constipation, even if you have bowel movements like these several times a day. So you should avoid anything that is likely to make you more constipated, eat a high-fiber diet, and ask your doctor whether bulking agents such as Metamucil, Fibercon, and Citrucel would help to make your bowel movements softer and more bulky. Bran (wheat bran, soy bran, or rice bran) may be helpful if you have abdominal pain plus constipation, but possibly not as effective (and not as palatable) as bulking agents. If one thing (bran, for example) has not improved your symptoms after three months, try something else (such as a bulking agent), as people differ in their responses to different types of fiber. Drink several pints of fluid a day while on a high-fiber diet.

Keep on the high-fiber diet for a few weeks, but if it appears to make your IBS worse, change to a low-fiber diet for about a month. While you are on a low-fiber diet it is important to take bulking agents such as Metamucil, Fibercon, or Citrucel to prevent constipation. If neither high-fiber nor low-fiber diets appear to work, try an exclusion diet to see if you have an intolerance to any particular food.

Number 4 is a normal, healthy bowel movement. If your stools are soft, bulky, and easy to pass, you should not be having serious problems. If you are, discuss them with your doctor. If your stools fit the description of numbers 6 or 7, this is diarrhea, even if you have only one bowel movement a day.

A high-fiber diet (especially if you take bran) will probably not do much good if your stools tend to be loose (types 5, 6, or 7) and may even make things worse. Instead try a low-fiber diet to give your gut a rest for a few weeks, especially if the problem started after a bout of holiday diarrhea. While on the low-fiber diet, it is important to take bulking agents such as Metamucil, Fibercon, or Citrucel to prevent constipation. If a low-fiber diet doesn't work, it may be that you have a food intolerance, in which case two weeks on an exclusion diet should help identify this. If an exclusion diet brings no relief, then it is highly likely that your IBS is not caused or triggered by problem foods, and you should look for some other cause, such as stress.

## Putting Your Diet into Practice

The high-fiber diet has been the traditional first line approach to Irritable Bowel Syndrome. It therefore seems a good way to start. If simple constipation is your main IBS symptom, a high-fiber diet will probably be effective and should reduce abdominal pain, too. But before we get into the specifics of that diet, let's take a look at what fiber is and why it's good for us.

## The Role of Fiber in Our Diet

You will remember that the large intestine, or colon, is a tube with muscular walls. The muscles of this tube work best if they can propel stools in a wavelike motion (by peristalsis) down to the storage depot of the rectum. The muscles move to compress the bowel contents, but if these are already compressed, hard, and dry, the natural activity of the bowel is largely wasted. Pressure builds up in the colon, causing pain and discomfort anywhere in the abdomen. Therefore, it's important to do everything you can to keep the contents of the bowel soft and bulky, and the simplest and most effective way to do this is to eat plenty of dietary fiber or roughage.

*Dietary fiber* is the material that makes up the cell walls of plants. It contains substances called cellulose, lignin, and polysaccharides. It is found in the skin, husks, and leaves of plants. If you were a rabbit or a cow or a caterpillar, you would eat large amounts of green material such as grass and leaves, and you would have in your gut the necessary enzymes to break them down in your digestive system, and it would do you a lot of good.

But we humans don't have these enzymes in our bodies and so can't digest dietary fiber. It just passes straight through us unchanged and undigested. Until quite recently, the received wisdom was that if it passed straight through then it couldn't be doing any good, so there wasn't much point in eating it. Now we know better.

Since dietary fiber is not digested and absorbed, it ends up in the large intestine much in the same condition as it entered the mouth. It helps bulks up stools so that they fill out the tubular bowel. This gives the bowel muscles something to work on, so pressure doesn't build up and cause pain and spasm. Dietary fiber also softens the stools, making them easy to pass. In addition, it allows the stools to hold more water in the bowel, so they become less dry. (Bacteria can break down fiber which is one reason why people who ingest psyllium do have an increase in bloating.)

Rural Africans eat large quantities of fruit and vegetables that are full of fiber. Researchers have found that the average rural African produces a large quantity of soft stools; that food passes through the gut in 36 hours or less; and that constipation, IBS, diverticular disease, and similar problems are almost unknown. (The average Westerner, by contrast, produces small quantities of fairly hard stools, and our food takes several days to pass through the gut.)

Fiber has other advantages unrelated to IBS: It fills you up more than highly refined foods do, so you eat less and may keep your weight down. It can help prevent diseases such as gall stones, diverticular disease, adult-onset diabetes, coronary heart disease, and blood clots following surgery. A high-fiber diet also reduces the risk of bowel and colon cancer, both of which are associated with the high-fat, low-fiber diet so common in our Western civilization. This is probably because fiber speeds up the passage of waste materials through the gut, which means that potentially harmful carcinogenic substances do not hang around long enough to do damage. Given its various merits, we now know that fiber's got to be a good thing.

## High-Fiber Diet

**Eat plenty of**

—Brown rice

—Green leafy vegetables (like spinach, broccoli, and kale)

—High-fiber breakfast cereals (like All-Bran)

—Potatoes in their skins

—Whole-grain bread

—Whole-grain flour

**Other good sources of fiber are**

—Apples

—Apricots

—Avocados

—Baked beans (though they may cause gas)

—Bananas

—Blackberries

—Black currants

—Brussels sprouts

—Cabbage

—Carrots

—Dates

—Figs

—Peas

—Prunes (stewed)

—Raspberries

—Red currants

—Rhubarb (though some find this makes their IBS worse)

—Spring greens

—Sweet corn (though some find this makes their IBS worse)

As mentioned before, it is important to drink plenty of fluids to ensure the fiber works well without drawing fluid from elsewhere in your body. If you are worried about your weight, keep to low-calorie fluids, such as skim milk (which keeps up your intake of calcium), water, and herb tea. Low-calorie canned drinks may contain additives that could upset your intestines.

Bran works well for many people, although some find it makes things worse. It reduces pressure in the large intestine, speeds up the passage of food through the digestive system, and absorbs water, thus making the stools softer, bulkier, and easier to pass. Take one tablespoon two or three times a day with meals, but be prepared to increase or decrease this amount according to the reaction you get. You will need to take less if you get abdominal pain and a bloated, uncomfortable feeling, and to take more if it doesn't appear to work. Stick with it for several weeks, since it can take up to three months to see how well it works.

## Low-Fiber Diet

Does a high-fiber diet make your IBS worse? Is diarrhea your main symptom? Or has an attack of "holiday tummy" started it off again? If so, you might benefit from a low-fiber diet.

The Gastroenterology Research Department of Addenbrooke's Hospital in Cambridge, England, recommend the following low-fiber diet to some of their IBS patients. (I am grateful to Dr. John Hunter for permission to reproduce it here.) Because a low-fiber diet contains very little dietary fiber (roughage) you may need to use a bulking agent such as Metamucil to prevent constipation. These bulk-forming laxatives are helpful, as opposed to stimulant laxatives.

## NOT RECOMMENDED

—Bran

—Brown pasta

—Brown rice

—Dried fruit (such as prunes, figs, apricots, currants, blackberries, raspberries)

—Fruit cakes

—Jam or marmalade with seeds and peel

—Nuts

—Oats

—Peas, beans, lentils, sweet corn, skins on potatoes

—Rye crackers

—Whole-grain cereals (such as bran flakes, muesli, Shredded Wheat)

—Whole-grain flour

## RECOMMENDED

### Cereals and breads

—Cakes and cookies made with white flour

—Corn flakes, Rice Krispies

—Croissants

—White bread

—White flour

—White pasta

—White rice

**Fruit**

—All fruits (skin removed when possible)

—Fruit juice

—Stewed or canned fruit

**Miscellaneous**

—Honey, syrup

—Ice cream

—Jelly, marmalade, and jam (without seeds or peel)

—Sugar

—Tea, coffee, cordial drinks

**Meat**

—All meat, fish, chicken

—Hamburgers

**Dairy**

—All milk, cheese, eggs, yogurt

—Butter, margarine

Be certain, however, that you eat a balanced diet that is not high in fat, sugar, or salt. All foods that are high in fiber should be avoided. These foods are mainly plant foods, and the most common are listed in the high-fiber diet.

Let us now suppose that neither the high-fiber diet nor the low-fiber diet has worked. What next? This is probably the time to consider whether you might have an intolerance to a particular food or foods. Food intolerance is a more likely possibility if diarrhea is your main IBS problem or if you have any allergic conditions such as asthma, some forms of eczema, hay fever, rhinitis, or urticaria.

Obviously, the first step is to conscientiously remove from your diet those foods that you know for certain disagree with you. Don't touch them for two weeks, and see whether your symptoms improve during this time. For many people this in itself will be enough. Then introduce the food in question in an average-size helping just to check whether it is indeed the villain; if you get no unpleasant reaction, you will at least know you can eat that food. If your symptoms return, cut that food out of your diet for up to six months before trying again. You may find that after giving your intestines a rest from it you can take it occasionally in small quantities without too much ill-effect.

However, it may be that you are really quite uncertain which foods are triggering your IBS. If that is so, a more systematic approach is needed.

## Exclusion Diet

Because there is no conclusive medical test for food intolerance, the "test" most commonly used to pinpoint problem foods is an exclusion diet. In its harshest form, patients exist on nothing but a few foods (say, lamb, pears and mineral water) for one to two weeks and then gradually introduce new foods, noting which foods cause an adverse reaction. Fortunately, exclusion diets such as that would only be used in the most extreme circumstances, with the patient under the close direction of a gastroenterologist and dietician.

Many gastroenterologists, general practitioners, and dieticians have devised their own exclusion diets as a means of finding which foods disagree with individual patients. The one that is used here has been developed by the Gastroenterology Research Department of Addenbrooke's Hospital in Cambridge. (I am grateful to Dr. John Hunter for permission to reprint it here.) It has been well tested and allows you to eat a wide range of foods to provide a healthy, balanced diet. When used under the direction of a competent clinician, it can resolve symptoms in about 50 percent of the patients.

If you have any doubts about your general state of health, you should ask your general practitioner whether it would be a good idea for you to try an exclusion diet. Or arrange to see a qualified dietician for advice. Be wary of undertaking any major change to your diet unsupervised, and don't use an exclusion diet on children except under medical supervision. If you have not had your IBS diagnosed by a doctor, this might be a good time to do it, to make sure you are not overlooking a more serious condition; in any case, you need to be sure you are treating the right thing.

The foods you can and can't eat are listed below. As the table implies, you can eat anything in the "allowed" column and nothing in the "not allowed" column. *It is important to keep strictly to the diet for two weeks.* It won't work if it is done half-heartedly. Having one of the forbidden foods even once could make it almost impossible to work out which foods disagree with you. But by taking time and commitment to do it properly there's a better-than-even chance you will improve your IBS beyond all recognition.

Keep a food diary during this period. Record the food you've eaten and the symptoms you've suffered.

| Food | Not Allowed | Allowed |
|------|-------------|---------|
| *Meat* | Beef, sausages | All other meats |
| | Hamburgers | Poultry and game |
| | Meat pies | Ham and bacon |
| *Fish* | Fish in batter or bread crumbs | White fish, fatty fish |
| | | Smoked fish, canned tuna |
| | | Canned sardines in soybean oil |
| | | Prawns |

| Food | Not Allowed | Allowed |
|------|-------------|---------|
| *Vegetables* | Potatoes<br>Onions<br>Canned vegetables<br>in sauce | All other fresh vegetables<br>Salad<br>Legumes (beans, peas,<br>lentils)<br>Canned vegetables |
| *Fruit* | Citrus fruit (oranges,<br>grapefruit, lemons) | All other fruit,<br>fresh or canned |
| *Cereals* | Wheat (bread, cakes,<br>cookies, pasta, noodles,<br>semolina, breakfast<br>cereals)<br>Sweet corn<br>Rye<br>Oats<br>Barley<br>Corn (corn flakes, corn<br>flour, custard powder) | Rice<br>Ground rice, rice flour<br>Rice Krispies, puffed<br>rice<br>Rice cakes<br>Arrowroot<br>Tapioca<br>Millet<br>Buckwheat<br>Quinoa |
| *Cooking Oils* | Corn oil<br>Vegetable oil | Sunflower oil<br>Canola oil, safflower oil<br>soybean oil, olive oil |
| *Dairy Products* | Cow's milk (all types)<br>Dried milk<br>Canned milk<br>Goat's milk<br>Butter<br>Cream<br>Margarine<br>Yogurt<br>Cheese<br>Eggs | Soy milk<br>Soy yogurt, soy ice cream<br>Tofu<br>Vegetable margarine |

| Food | Not Allowed | Allowed |
|------|-------------|---------|
| *Beverages* | Tea (caffeinated or decaffeinated) | Herbal teas, (rose hips, peppermint, chamomile) |
| | Coffee (caffeinated or decaffeinated) | Fresh fruit juices, (apple, pineapple, tomato, grape) |
| | Fruit shakes | Mineral water |
| | Canned drinks | |
| | Orange juice | |
| | Grapefruit juice | |
| | Lemon juice | |
| | Alcohol | |
| | Tap water | |
| *Miscellaneous* | Marmalade, jams containing preservatives and colors | Pure fruit spread |
| | | Homemade jam |
| | Mustard | Salt, herbs, black pepper |
| | Yeast | Spices in moderation |
| | Yeast extract | Sugar, honey |
| | Gravy mixes | Brown rice miso |
| | Vinegar | Gravy browning containing caramel and salt only |
| | Nuts | Dried fruit (wash first) |
| | Baking powder containing wheat | Gluten-free baking powder |
| | Chocolate | Dried banana, coconut, sunflower seeds |

The list of foods in the "not allowed" column may seem rather daunting at first, but there is such a good range of foods in the "allowed" column that you shouldn't have much difficulty following this diet for two weeks. But in case you feel there is nothing left to eat, here is a list of possible meals for one week (wheat-free and dairy-free recipes are given at the end of this chapter for foods marked with a star [❂]):

**Breakfast**

—Homemade muesli⊙

—Stewed fruit (apples, apricots, prunes) with or without goat's milk or yogurt, and sweetened with honey

—Rice crackers, with nondairy spread and jam or honey

—Rice Krispies (or any cereal that does not contain wheat, corn, oats, or rye) with a milk substitute or fruit juice

—Apple, pineapple, or tomato juice

—Herb tea

**Lunch and Dinner**

*Day 1*

—Lunch: cauliflower in cheese sauce⊙; raw apple

—Dinner: avocado salad with apple and beet root in yogurt dressing⊙; banana jello⊙

*Day 2*

—Lunch: buckwheat croquettes⊙ with vegetables; melon

—Dinner: grilled trout with mushrooms and peas; baked pears with honey

*Day 3*

—Lunch: homemade soup⊙; bananas

—Dinner: grilled lamb's liver; mushrooms, carrots, cauliflower; baked apple stuffed with grapes and honey

*Day 4*

—Lunch: green pepper stuffed with rice and mushrooms; mixed dried fruit soaked overnight in apple juice

—Dinner: leeks, cauliflower, celery, zucchini, string beans (according to season) in cheese sauce⊙; fresh fruit (not citrus)

*Day 5*

—Lunch: lentil rissoles (fritters) (taste better if made the day before); fresh fruit (not citrus)

—Dinner: grilled lamb chops and vegetables (not potatoes, onions, cabbage or sweet corn); rice pudding❂

*Day 6*

—Lunch: grilled chicken (hot or cold) with salad of apple, zucchini, cauliflower or cucumber; stewed fruit

—Dinner: stir-fry of sprouting vegetables with any other vegetables (except potatoes, cabbage, onions, or sweet corn) and flavored with tamari (a wheat-free soy sauce); baked bananas (cooked with honey and nondairy margarine)

*Day 7*

—Lunch: grilled white fish with vegetables; fresh fruit (not citrus)

—Dinner: risotto with spinach, leftover chicken, and any other vegetables; fresh fruit salad (with no citrus fruits)

With any luck you will feel that spending two weeks on an exclusion diet is not impossible and that you can eat varied, interesting meals. However, be prepared that the first few days on the exclusion diet may be unpleasant as your body gets used to being without the foods it has had regularly. This is usually a good sign. You should feel much better in about a week, so stick with the diet, and don't be tempted to give up if you feel worse at the very beginning. If you continue to feel worse after about a week, it could be that a new replacement food is the culprit, especially if you are eating a lot of it to substitute for a food in the "not allowed" column. If this happens, you will need to cut out any new food that you have introduced into your diet.

In addition to the foods in the "not allowed" column, exclude any foods that you know disagree with you. With any luck, you will only have to go without them for the two weeks you are on the diet, and there are lots of acceptable alternatives. (See Appendix.)

Eat as wide a variety as possible from the foods in the "allowed" column to ensure a healthy, balanced diet. Keep an accurate diary of everything you eat and of any symptoms you have. Be sure to note times when the symptoms occur. Any symptoms you notice will probably have been caused by one of the foods eaten in the previous twenty-four hours, and this should help you pinpoint the source of the trouble.

You should see a steady improvement in your IBS symptoms during the second week; if this happens, you can gradually start to reintroduce new foods, in the following order:

| | |
|---|---|
| 1. Tap water | 9. Eggs |
| 2. Potatoes | 10. Oats |
| 3. Cow's milk | 11. Coffee |
| 4. Yeast | 12. Chocolate |
| 5. Tea | 13. Barley |
| 6. Rye | 14. Citrus fruits |
| 7. Butter | 15. Corn |
| 8. Onions | 16. Cow's cheese |
| 17. White wine | 21. Wheat |
| 18. Shellfish | 22. Nuts |
| 19. Cow's yogurt | 23. Preservatives |
| 20. Vinegar | 24. Processed foods |

Introduce these new foods at the rate of one every two days. Eat a good-sized portion of it, not just a tiny nibble. During this time continue to keep your diary of everything you eat, the symptoms you get, and when. Only by doing this will you know which newly introduced food is the cause of your symptoms. If you have a bad reaction to something, flush out your digestive system by drinking plenty of water (adding a little bicarbonate of soda helps).

When you have reintroduced all the foods, go back and test them again to be sure. If only one or two less common foods are troubling you, this should be no problem, because there are acceptable substitutes for almost everything. But if you now find that many foods trigger your symptoms, and especially if basic foods like wheat and dairy products are among them, arrange to see a dietician to make sure the diet you must follow in the future will be nutritionally adequate.

Having found that foods disagree with you, keep off them for about six months, to give your digestive system a complete rest from them. Then try again after another six months. If the time comes when that food causes no reaction, eat it once a week to begin with, then perhaps twice a week, but never every day. You will have to be your own judge about how often you can eat it.

If after two weeks on the exclusion diet you are not feeling considerably better, food intolerance is probably not the cause of your IBS symptoms. In this case, see if your doctor has any other treatment to offer or consider some form of alternative therapy such as osteopathy, homeopathy, acupuncture, medical herbalism, or hypnotherapy.

If you get a lot of pain after meals, try a low-fat diet; but don't cut out fats altogether, because they are important for the correct working of the body. Choose foods marked "low-fat" and select lean cuts of low-fat meats such as chicken, turkey, and rabbit; avoid higher-fat fish such as mackerel and herring.

## Recipes for Dishes Marked with Star (✪)

### BANANA JELLO

Sprinkle a packet of gelatin on 3 fl. oz. of heated apple juice and stir until dissolved. Make up to 1 pint with more apple juice. Add sliced bananas. Leave to set. (Other fruits can be used to give variety.)

## BUCKWHEAT CROQUETTES

Cook 6 oz. buckwheat in twice its own volume of water until the water has been absorbed and the buckwheat is soft; drain and cool. Add finely chopped celery, carrots, and/or leeks; 1 oz. soy flour; seasoning; and herbs. Shape into rounds a half-inch thick and fry or bake on both sides until cooked.

## CHEESE SAUCE

Melt 1 oz. nondairy margarine; blend in 1 oz. soy flour, cook for 1 minute, then slowly mix in 10 fl. oz. soy milk, stirring all the time with a wooden spoon. When thoroughly blended, add 2 to 3 oz. nondairy cheese (or any other flavoring that you prefer) and stir until melted.

## HOMEMADE SOUP

Cook together plenty of suitable chopped or shredded vegetables and a cup of red lentils, without salt, until soft. Mix them all in a blender. Add seasoning and water until it has a souplike consistency. If you have a pressure cooker, soup can be made very quickly.

## MUESLI

Mix together buckwheat (no relation to wheat, despite its name) or millet with dried fruits such as apricots, raisins, grapes, and chopped apple. Serve with a milk substitute (such as soy milk) and honey. Some other recipes for wheat-free muesli are on pages 208–209.

## RICE PUDDING

Sprinkle 3 oz. flaked rice onto 1 pint of nearly boiling milk substitute. Simmer for 10 to 15 minutes (or according to directions on packet). Sweeten with honey and serve alone or with stewed fruit.

## YOGURT DRESSING

Mix goat's milk yogurt with chopped mint, chives, garlic, and seasoning (unless you know that any of these disagree with you, in which case you should use your closest substitute).

# Not Just What You Eat, But How

If you have IBS, it is quite likely that at least part of your life is tense and stressful. Yet it is important to be emotionally relaxed when eating, or else your IBS gets worse. Try to follow these rules:

—Don't eat when you are tense, angry, or anxious.

—Allow plenty of time for each meal.

—Don't eat standing up, "on the run," or perched on a stool—sit down on a chair.

—"Grazing" (eating as you move about) may be fashionable, but it does the digestive system no good at all.

—Take time to shop for and prepare wholesome foods.

—Try not to swallow air while you are eating.

—Decide in advance how much you are going to eat, and don't be tempted to eat more.

—Stop eating as soon as you feel full.

—Cut down on rich food.

—Allow two to three hours between your last meal and bedtime.

Think carefully before you embark on a crash diet. Many people can trace their IBS back to such a diet, possibly due to a sudden drop in fiber and to eating a different range of foods. Crash dieting can induce constipation, which in itself can cause IBS symptoms and may then be followed by diarrhea.

There are now well-recognized guidelines for more nutritious eating, so try to follow them. For example:

—Trim excess fat off meat before cooking.

—Grill rather than fry.

—Avoid deep-fat frying.

—Eat fresh fruits and vegetables rather than canned, frozen, or processed.

—Eat the skins of boiled or baked potatoes.

—Use as little salt as possible in cooking and at the table.

—Eat whole grains and whole-grain breads and pastas; avoid white rice and white-flour products unless otherwise directed.

—Have some leafy green vegetables every day.

—Substitute fresh food for processed food wherever possible.

Simply following these guidelines could work wonders for your IBS, especially if you are bothered by constipation and abdominal pain; but it is also important to eat in a calm, relaxed way, giving your digestive system the opportunity to work properly.

Give time, too, to choosing what you eat. If you don't think about this in advance, you will probably find it is time for the next meal and you haven't got anything to eat; so you rush to the nearest shop and choose something that you can cook and eat in no time at all—and then wonder why you have a stomach ache. It is a good idea to sit down quietly for about twenty minutes a week and write down on paper what you will have for each meal. Perhaps you will choose some of the recipes in later chapters or from any book on good healthy eating. When you have decided what you will have for each meal, make a shopping list and buy everything all at once—that way you will always have something good and nutritious in the house and won't be tempted to eat junk food because you are in a hurry.

No matter what you are cutting out from your diet, you should have no difficulty finding acceptable alternatives. Here are some ideas for creative eating on a restricted diet:

—Legumes (lentils, beans, and so on) are a useful, low-cost, high-protein alternative to meat and can be made into numerous delicious meals. Get into the habit of putting some to soak in a bowl or saucepan at bedtime or before you go to work, so they are ready to cook when you need them.

—Rice cakes are a good alternative to bread and crackers if you can't eat wheat.

—You can make rice flour by grinding rice very finely, but it cooks rather differently from wheat flour, so experiment with it first.

—Have you tried tofu? Gram for gram, it is the cheapest and richest source or protein available except for eggs (which are high in cholesterol). Tofu is made from soybeans, is low in salt and saturated fat and free from cholesterol. Although almost tasteless in itself, it absorbs the flavors of other ingredients. It is available in most health food stores and supermarkets and is highly nutritious—it's also an ideal diet food.

Handle tofu gently; when you get it home, unwrap it and put it in the fridge in a bowl of water, completely covered so it doesn't absorb other flavors. Change the water daily. It will keep fresh for about a week from the day it was made.

—Nowadays, we expect foods to keep for weeks or even months, but this is usually only possible by adding preservatives and other additives that may aggravate your IBS. So be prepared to accept more natural storage times.

If you are eating a restricted diet, you may be considering taking dietary supplements (such as vitamin pills) to make up for the perceived nutritional shortfall in your diet. If you do not eat wheat products, you may become deficient in B-group vitamins, and if you do not eat dairy products, you will need to get enough calcium from somewhere, so supplements may be the answer for you. If in doubt, ask your doctor.

Unfortunately, many people who live life in the fast lane feel that it is enough to eat a totally inadequate diet and then compensate by taking vitamins, minerals, and other supplements in the forms of pills, potions, and powders. Many use dietary supplements as a substitute for sensible living. Instead of reducing the stress in their lives they take "stress-reducing pills"; instead of tackling the causes of insomnia they take sleeping pills; instead of eating plenty of roughage and worrying less about minor constipation they take laxatives. Your IBS may well have been caused by the life you lead, and it is not possible to prevent or reverse the ravages of a bad lifestyle with a pill. Nutrition by pills is not nutrition; we should not deceive ourselves that it is.

## Ideas and Recipes for Healthy Living

One of the main things your irritable bowel needs is good, healthy food eaten in a calm, leisurely way. Anything else is asking for trouble. Whether you are a stressed-out businessperson, a hassled parent, or a working person in a hurry, the time you spend planning, cooking, and eating wholesome, sensible food will be a worthwhile investment. The alternative is all the awful symptoms of Irritable Bowel Syndrome.

"Wholesome, sensible food" is not the kiss of death. You can forget all about boiled fish, gruel, and bread and milk. Just flipping through the recipes that follow should convince you that eating to please your irritable bowel can be quick, interesting, and inexpensive.

Many of the recipes in this chapter are wheat-free, since this is a more difficult diet to follow, and there are fewer cookbooks available. In the section on bread, dough, cakes, and cookies, wheat-free recipes are marked WF. However, the majority of IBS sufferers should be thinking less about a wheat-free diet and more about a high-fiber diet, so unless you know that you must avoid wheat you should be using whole grain bread and whole grain flour rather than wheat-free bread and flour. There are many high-fiber diet cookbooks around—your local library or bookstores will probably have several.

If wheat disagrees with you, you can choose to eat it just occasionally or in very small quantities in the hope that your gut can cope with it or use a recipe with a wheat-free flour such as quinoa, or spelt.

If dairy products disagree with you, you can choose to eat them occasionally or in very small quantities, as with wheat. Or you can use substitutes such as soy milk instead of animal milk and nondairy spreads instead of ordinary butter and margarine. Use these according to how your digestive systems reacts to dairy products.

If you have problems with other foods (such as onions, citrus fruits, chocolates, or potatoes, for example), you should check each recipe carefully and either leave out the offending food or choose a different recipe. Also, some recipes call for prepared items, such as bouillon cubes, for convenience. Do check that they don't contain any ingredients that give you problems.

## Breakfast

Do you grab a cup of coffee some time between getting up and starting the day and call it "breakfast"? Do you sit at the breakfast bar, drinking coffee with one hand and shaving or applying makeup with the other? Do you get up about five minutes before you have to leave for work? Are you in such a rush to get the children off to school that you don't have any time to sit down and relax? If so, then it's hardly surprising you have Irritable Bowel Syndrome!

It really needn't be like this. As you have already read, it is important to allow plenty of time at the start of the day for a relaxed breakfast and then to disappear to the toilet for ten minutes or more to make sure you do not get constipated. The "bowel-emptying" message is strongest after meals, particularly first thing in the morning, and you ignore it at your own peril. It is highly likely that your irritable bowel is caused by the life you lead, so the start of the day is a good time to begin doing things differently.

Get up early enough to allow yourself plenty of time in the morning. Always eat a good breakfast; sit down at the table in a quiet, leisurely way; reading a morning paper or magazine is a good way to prolong breakfast. If coffee disagrees with you, drink black tea, herb tea, or other alternatives; you'll quickly get used to them.

If citrus fruits and juices disagree with you, try apple juice, tomato juice, pineapple juice, and so on.

Provided you are not sensitive to wheat or on a low-fiber diet, eat a high-fiber cereal, followed by whole grain toast and perhaps some stewed fruit such as apricots or prunes.

## MUESLI

The following are three recipes for wheat-free muesli. You can add or eliminate ingredients according to taste. Mix together dry ingredients and keep in a food storage jar. At bedtime, put some of the dry mixture in a cereal bowl, cover with water or apple juice, and leave to soak overnight. At breakfast serve the muesli with fresh fruit, dried fruit, and/or yogurt.

6 tablespoons flaked millet WF

4 tablespoons flaked rice

2 tablespoons chopped nuts

1 teaspoon chopped dried fruit

1 teaspoon toasted sesame seeds

—OR—

4 tablespoons flaked rice WF

4 tablespoons oatmeal

1 tablespoon sunflower seeds

1 tablespoon chopped nuts

1 tablespoon raisins, grapes, or currants

—OR—

4 tablespoons of any of the following (or a mixture): medi-
um oatmeal, rolled oats, barley flakes, millet flakes, rye
flakes; add 1 tablespoon of soy or rice bran WF

You can also add any of the following to muesli: sesame seeds, sunflower seeds, dried fruit (such as dates, apricots, raisins, peaches),
nuts (walnuts, hazelnuts, almonds, cashews, brazils, and so on),
and any fresh fruit that doesn't disagree with you.

It is worth visiting the store to buy the basic ingredients once
every week or so and spending a few minutes mixing them together. Experiment with small quantities, until you find the combination you like, then make up a large quantity and keep it in a food
storage jar.

### STEWED FRUIT

Put some dried fruit (apricots, prunes, pears, raisins, for example)
in a bowl covered with plenty of water (or cold tea) and leave to
soak for several hours until soft. You can speed the process up by
bringing the water gently to a boil first. Add sugar as necessary.
Serve hot or cold.

### EGGS

These can be boiled, poached, baked, or scrambled. (Be sure to
cook them thoroughly to kill salmonella bacteria.)

## Midday Meal at Work

How has your day gone so far? Did you get up in a rush? Miss breakfast? Dash out of the house to stand in an overcrowded train or bus?
Or perhaps to sit in a traffic jam tapping your fingers impatiently on
the steering wheel while you talk on the car phone or plan the day's
work? Have you just finished the first of many cups of coffee while
doing a hundred other things? Not a good start to the day!

And now it's somewhere between noon and 2 p.m.—time for
something to eat. What will you have? A bag of chips? A cigarette

and a cup of coffee? A chocolate bar? After all, you're so busy you haven't time to eat properly, have you? You have time to sit in traffic jams, work late, or slump in front of the television, but eating, shopping, cooking? Of course not. And then you wonder why your gut acts up!

Ultimately, of course, the choice is yours. As you have already read, you can decide whether to continue with the very lifestyle that provokes your irritable bowel, or you can make a few changes here and there and, with luck, bring it under your control. Reducing stress is one important way; looking at how and what you eat is another.

The midday meal can be an obvious problem. You may have to eat a lot of business lunches or spend your lunch hour rushing around doing the family shopping; you may feel you want to go out to the takeout place with your colleagues, or you may not like the food in the cafeteria. And if, on top of all this, certain foods disagree with you, any form of eating out can be stressful. Will the beef stroganoff have onions in it? Does the pizza crust have a wheat base? Will the sauce on the lasagna contain milk?

Consider too all the additives that are part and parcel of instant food: colorings, emulsifiers, stabilizers, thickeners, preservatives, antioxidants, flavor enhancers, and flavorings. Very few restaurants and even fewer takeout places and cafeterias make their food entirely from scratch; nearly all use catering-quality foods in one form or another, which tend to be high in additives.

If you can make a brown-bag lunch that is easy to shop for and simple to make, you can avoid these problems. It is obviously more trouble to do this, but if it eases your irritable bowel, you may decide it is worth it.

Here are a collection of ideas to make it easy for you to eat wholesome foods in the middle of the day. Many of them require access to a microwave or conventional oven in order to reheat them, but more and more firms and offices now have a microwave. If yours doesn't, perhaps you could persuade your boss that it would be a good investment. The cost would be comparatively small, it would take up very little space, and by encouraging employees to eat nutritiously in the middle of the day the organization is investing in their health, which is a financially (and morally) sound thing to do.

Even if you cannot use an oven or microwave, you will still find plenty of ideas here for a quick, easy, and nutritionally healthy midday meal.

—Invest in some suitable containers: a thermos, a lunch box, some plastic bowls with lids, some containers for reheating food in a microwave, or anything else you might need to take food to work and cook and eat it there.

—To save time in the morning, most snacks can be made the previous night, wrapped in cling wrap or put in a plastic container, and kept in the fridge. Salads can also be loosely packed in plastic bags.

—There is more to a packed lunch than a curled-up ham sandwich. Try filling a pocket of pita bread or a French roll. Whatever you use, put in plenty of filling.

—To save yourself time and effort, make enough for two or three meals and freeze what you don't use for another day. Or make a basic meal, then vary it slightly for the next two or three days.

—Eat plenty of fruit, fresh or dried.

—Try to plan a whole week's lunchtime menus—it's a lot less hassle than having to think about it each day. Also, by buying enough for the whole week you avoid running short and having to fall back on junk food. You've got to think about it some time, but one long "think" is a lot easier than five short ones!

—Each week buy a few fillings for sandwiches or pita bread and rotate them in combination. You could try

| | |
|---|---|
| Apple (sliced) | Hummus |
| Bean sprouts | Lentils (mashed, cooked) |
| Carrots (grated) | Lunchmeat (lean) |
| Celery (finely chopped) | Mushrooms |
| Cheese (grated) | Sardines |
| Cottage cheese | Tomatoes |
| Cucumber | Tuna |
| Dried figs or apricots | Watercress |
| Eggs (hard-boiled | Zucchini (sliced) |
|     or scrambled) | Anything else you'd like |

—If you can't eat wheat, take some rice cakes to work instead of bread or biscuits; or make your own bread, crackers, chapatis, and so on from the recipes on pages 227–33.

—Baked potatoes are cheap, filling, and nutritious and can easily be filled at home and taken to work, although you will need a microwave to heat them up. Possible fillings are

| | |
|---|---|
| Bacon | Lettuce or cabbage (sliced) |
| Carrot (grated) | Mushrooms |
| Cheese | Prawns |
| Chicken | Tomato and onion |
| Coleslaw (homemade) | Tuna |
| Cucumber | Turkey |
| Egg (scrambled) | Yogurt |
| Egg (with mayonnaise) | Anything else, including |
| Ham |     leftovers |

—If you can tolerate just a little wheat, rye crackers may suit you.

—Buy an empty pie crust (most supermarkets sell them) and fill it with any combinations of fillings you like, possibly bound together with a cheese sauce, and take a slice to work. Freeze the rest or, if you don't have a freezer, fill the pie crust with different fillings in two or three segments and cut each segment when you need it. It will keep for three or four days in a fridge.

—It's very easy to make your own yogurt. Put into a bowl one tablespoon of plain yogurt (it doesn't have to be "live" yogurt, as long as it has no additives such as preservatives). Heat one pint of milk to 125°F and pour carefully onto the yogurt in the bowl. Stir very gently, cover with a plate, and leave in a warm place overnight. By morning it should have set and have a thin layer of liquid on the top. Drain off the liquid. Now you can put some into a plastic bowl with a lid and take it to work. Add anything you like, such as

| | |
|---|---|
| Apple or pear (finely chopped) | Honey |
| Apricots (chopped, dried) | Mandarin oranges |
| Banana (mashed) | Prunes (chopped) |
| Hazelnuts | Raspberries |

—Set aside a tablespoon of this yogurt as the starter for the next batch you make. You can also add it to main dishes, use it as the base of delicious drinks, or as a substitute for oil in salad dressings. Store it in the fridge.

—Take to work one or more of the salads on pages 225–26.

—Pizza is quick and easy to make and convenient to take to work. Some supermarkets sell plain pizza bases for you to add your own ingredients.

—Crêpes, too, make a good midday meal and can be filled with anything you like. Basic recipes are on pages 222–23. Savory crêpes usually need to be heated.

—Hummus is high in protein, easy to make, and can be used as part of a salad, or as a basic filling in sandwiches or pita bread. The recipe is on pages 226–27.

—To cut down on coffee, keep some fruit juice or some herb teabags at work. Also keep some herb teabags in your pocket or bag for when you are visiting.

—Take some fruit to work every day.

—Some suggestions for instant snacks are

| | |
|---|---|
| Cashew nuts | Potato chips (without |
| Coconut (desiccated) | additives) |
| Fruit (dried) | Pumpkin seeds |
| Pistachio nuts | Sesame seed bars |
| Popcorn | Sunflower seeds |

—Having gone to the trouble of planning, buying, and preparing your midday meal, don't destroy the benefit by gobbling it down as you rush from A to B. Find a quiet place and sit down in a comfortable chair. Give yourself permission to take time off to eat in peace and digest your meal.

## Recipes

### SOUPS

Homemade soups are nutritious, easy to make, and ideal to take to work in a thermos. Soups containing vegetables are a good source of dietary fiber (roughage).

Even if you can't be bothered to make a meal some evenings, a bowl of homemade soup with a hunk of thick bread is filling, healthy, and cheap. Sprinkle grated cheese on it and have some fresh fruit to follow. What could be more wholesome and delicious?

It's not difficult to get into the habit of making soup regularly, and each batch will last a while if kept in the fridge or frozen for another day. If you have an oven or microwave at work, take the soup with you cold; if not, heat it up before you leave home and keep it hot in a thermos.

Some of the recipes in this chapter do not give specific quantities—it's up to you to choose how much of each vegetable you like; even where quantities are given, they are meant as guidance. You can usually be as flexible as you like and make variations according to your taste and what is available. Also, you can make the soup thick or thin according to how much water or stock you add; there's nothing to stop you making soups so thick you can eat them with a fork! If you have a blender or food processor, it's easier to make "creamed" soups than having to force the ingredients through a sieve; and a pressure cooker will greatly reduce the cooking time if you are using vegetables that take longer to cook, like parsnips, potatoes, and legumes. Even if you have neither of these, you can still make delicious, wholesome soups.

You can use any vegetables, in any combination. If you cream the soup in a blender or food processor, adding lentils (or other legumes) or potatoes will thicken it, while adding more water or stock will make it thinner. (If using lentils, add salt *after* they are cooked, or they will take ages to soften). Once you have followed a few recipes you will quickly see how to make your own soups any way you like them.

## Bean and Tomato Soup

*8 oz. lima beans or 1 can of lima beans or 1 can red kidney beans*
*2 onions*
*oil, butter, or margarine*
*1 can of tomatoes*

If using dried lima beans, soak them overnight. Cook onions in saucepan in oil, butter, or margarine. Add tomatoes, beans, and about 3½ cups water. Simmer very gently until beans are tender (about 10 minutes if using canned beans; longer if using fresh). Season as necessary.

## Celery Soup

*1 bunch of celery, washed and chopped*
*½ cup milk*
*2 oz. red lentils*
*1 cup water*
*1 clove garlic, crushed*

Put all the ingredients into a saucepan and simmer until soft. Liquefy in a blender and add seasoning as necessary.

## Chicken Noodle Soup

*1 onion*
*1 clove garlic*
*2 chicken joints, cut into pieces*
*2 oz. Chinese-style noodles*
*6 oz. Chinese cabbage, chopped*

Fry the onion and garlic in a saucepan until transparent. Add the pieces of chicken and cover with water. Bring to a boil and season with salt and pepper. Cover and simmer for about 1 hour. Remove the chicken bones and skin and continue boiling to reduce the liquid by about half. Add the noodles and cabbage, simmer for a few minutes, and serve.

## Cream of Carrot Soup

*1 lb. carrots, thinly sliced*
*½ lb. tomatoes (chopped), or 12 oz. canned*
*3½ cups stock*
*1 cup milk*
*2 oz. butter or margarine*
*chopped parsley*

Melt the butter in a saucepan and cook carrots gently for a few minutes, stirring occasionally. Add tomatoes and cook for another few minutes. Pour in the stock, season as necessary, and simmer until the carrots are soft (about 45 minutes). Liquefy in a blender. Add milk and reheat gently. Serve sprinkled with chopped parsley.

## Leek and Carrot Soup

*2 large carrots, diced*
*4 leeks, chopped*
*1 oz. butter or margarine*
*3½ cups stock or water*
*chopped parsley*

Sauté leeks and carrots together in butter or margarine in a saucepan until slightly browned. Add stock or water, cover pan, and cook gently for 30 to 40 minutes until vegetables are cooked. Serve as it is for a thin soup or liquefy for a thick soup. Sprinkle with chopped parsley.

## Lentil Soup

*1 cup red lentils*
*2 small onions*
*1 clove garlic, crushed or chopped*
*salt and seasonings to taste*
*3½ cups water*
*any leftover cooked, chopped potatoes, carrots, or celery (optional)*

Heat the oil in a saucepan. Cook the finely chopped onions and garlic in the oil until soft. Add the lentils and water and bring to a boil. Simmer until lentils are soft (about 20 to 30 minutes), then add seasoning and chopped vegetables. Continue cooking until vegetables are tender.

## Onion Soup

*4 large onions, finely sliced*
*2 oz. butter or margarine*
*3½ cups strong-flavored stock*

Melt the butter in a saucepan and fry the onions until they become translucent. Pour in the stock and bring to a boil. Season as necessary and simmer gently for about 45 minutes.

## Oxtail Soup

*1 oxtail (usually bought from butcher ready cut-up and bound)*
*butter or oil*
*onions*
*stock*

Cook oxtail in the oven for an hour or two. (It is more economical to put it in a warm oven in a casserole dish and cook it on the bottom rack while something else is cooking.) Remove the oxtail and skim off the fat when cool. Fry onions in butter or oil until they turn a light brown, add the oxtail and stock, and cook together for about 15 minutes. Season as necessary. (Pressure cooking cuts down cooking time considerably.)

## Potato–Leek Soup

*1 oz. butter or margarine*
*3 leeks, washed and sliced*
*3 large potatoes, peeled and chopped*
*1 cube of chicken or vegetable stock*
*3½ cups water*

Melt the butter in a saucepan and fry the leeks and potatoes lightly with the lid on the pan for about 20 minutes. Dissolve the stock cube in some boiling water, then add more water to make about 3½ cups. Simmer for another 10 minutes or until cooked. Season as necessary.

MAIN DISHES

The recipes in this section are just a tiny selection of what you could eat at a main meal. They are inexpensive, easy to shop for, quick to prepare, and nutritious. Most of them have a good fiber content. There is nothing magical about them—you can adapt them according to your preferences and to what's in your kitchen cupboard.

## Cheesy Leeks

(This recipe also works with other vegetables.)

*at least 4 leeks*
*1 oz. butter or margarine*
*1 oz. flour*
*1 cup milk*
*grated cheese*
*Worcestershire sauce (optional)*

Wash the leeks (or other vegetables), cut them into fairly large portions, and place in an ovenproof dish. Then make the cheese sauce: melt butter or margarine in a saucepan, stir in flour until it makes a paste, and slowly add milk, stirring until quite smooth. Add enough grated cheese to give a good flavor and add a few drops of Worcestershire sauce (optional). Pour sauce over vegetables, sprinkle some more grated cheese on top, and bake for about 30 minutes at 350°F.

## Chicken Parcels
### (Serves 1)

*1 chicken portion*
*lemon and thyme stuffing (packaged)*
*1 large potato*
*1 or 2 wide strips of bacon*

Make up a small quantity of lemon and thyme stuffing (about 1 to 2 tablespoons per person) and spread over chicken portion. Wrap a strip of bacon around it. Cut potato in half lengthwise and place one half on each side of the chicken. Sprinkle with salt and pepper. Wrap all rounds with foil, turn over edges of foil to seal well, and bake for about an hour at 350°F.

## Quick Chicken Casserole
### (Serves 1)

*1 chicken portion*
*1 can of mushroom soup*
*sliced vegetables, such as carrots, zucchini, celery, or leeks*
*2 lemon wedges*

Place chicken portions in casserole dish and cover with mushroom soup and sliced vegetables. Add lemon wedges. Cook for about 30 to 40 minutes at 350°F. Remove lemon before serving.

### PASTA

Pasta is cheap, nutritious, and easy to prepare. Whole-wheat pasta is higher in fiber than ordinary (egg) pasta. Allow 3 to 4 oz. per person, more if you are very hungry. Pasta comes in a wide range of shapes, and you can serve it with any number of different sauces. Cooking times differ according to the make and variety, so check the package for instructions.

Some ideas for pasta sauce are

—onion and tomato

—mushroom and tomato

—mushroom, garlic, and yogurt

—tuna fish and mushroom

—chicken liver and tomato

—tomato and herbs

—prawn and tomato

Pasta also makes a very good salad. Allow about 2 oz. per person and add anything you like, with a light dressing:

—cubes of cheese

—pieces of tuna fish

—red, green, and yellow peppers

—leftover cold meats

—sliced zucchini

—thinly sliced leeks

—chopped hard-boiled eggs

—mushrooms, cooked or raw

—nuts

—chopped oranges or apples

If you can't eat wheat, your local supermarket or health food store may stock wheat-free pasta.

### RICE

Rice is one of the few foods that seems to disagree with almost nobody. Allow about 3 oz. per person for a main dish and about 2 oz. per person for a salad.

## Rice Salad

Cook the rice according to the instructions on the packet and allow it to cool. While it is still warm, fluff it up with a fork if it looks like it is sticking together. When cold you can add almost anything you want to it, with or without a dressing.

## Simple Risotto

(This recipe uses white rice; if using brown rice, use more liquid and allow a longer cooking time.)

*1 onion, chopped*
*butter, margarine, or oil*
*4 oz. rice*

*2 oz. grated cheese*

*1½ cups chicken stock, or 1 chicken stock cube dissolved in about 1½
cups boiling water*

*a handful of currants*

*about 3 oz. leftover cooked chicken or ham, diced*

Fry the onion lightly in the butter, margarine, or oil until translucent. Stir in the rice and cook for a few minutes. Carefully add the stock and simmer gently until all the liquid has been absorbed and the rice is just cooked (white rice takes 15 to 20 minutes; brown rice usually takes 30 to 40 minutes). Add the currants, diced meat, and grated cheese, mix quickly together, heat through for about 5 minutes, and serve at once.

## CRÊPES

You can eat crêpes many ways: on their own, stuffed with meats or vegetables, covered with sauce, or dry, as you wish.

## Wheat Crêpes
### A recipe for those who can eat wheat:

*4 oz. plain flour*

*a pinch of salt*

*2 eggs*

*1 cup milk (You can replace 2 to 3 oz. of the milk with water if you
prefer*

*2 tablespoons melted butter or margarine*

Sift the flour and salt into a mixing bowl. Make a well in the middle and break the eggs into it. Beat well, gradually incorporating the flour into the eggs. Add the milk (or milk and water) and beat well until you have a nice, smooth mixture; lumps will disappear as you continue beating. (The mixture should have the consistency of thin cream.) Put a very small pat of butter or margarine into a frying pan and allow it to thinly cover the whole base of the pan. Pour into the pan about three-quarters of a ladleful (about 2 tablespoons) of the batter mixture, swirl the pan around quickly so that the mixture quickly and evenly spreads over the base of the pan, and cook for about a minute on each side. When the crêpe is cooked it should flip easily. You may find the first crêpe is not too successful, but the rest should be fine.

## Wheat-free Crêpes
### Two crêpe recipes for those who can't eat wheat:

*2 oz. gluten-free flour WF*
*¼ teaspoon wheat-free baking powder*
*1 egg*
*½ cup skim milk*

Put the flour into a bowl with the egg and mix to a stiff paste. Add the milk, a little at a time, beating it in after each addition. Beat well and it is ready to use.

—OR—

*1 oz. buckwheat WF*
*1 oz. rice flour*
*2 oz. gluten-free cornmeal*
*1 egg*
*½ cup milk*

Mix the buckwheat and rice flour together in a bowl with a little salt. Add the egg and milk, stir well, and leave to stand for 15 minutes. Then stir again, and it is ready to use.

## STUFFED VEGETABLES

You can stuff bell peppers, squash, or even giant mushrooms. For peppers, slice them lengthwise, remove the seeds, and blanch in boiling water for about 2 minutes to reduce the strong taste. For squash, cut lengthwise and bake for 30 minutes or until squash is partly done. Fill with a stuffing of any combinations of

*rice*
*diced cooked chicken or ham*
*nuts*
*mushrooms*
*peas*

*tuna*

*finely chopped leeks and celery*

*leftovers*

Place in a well-greased oven dish, cover, and cook until tender.

## FISH

Fish is a much-underrated dish. It is quick and easy to prepare and most nutritious. It can be grilled, baked, poached, or cooked in foil. Choose fresh fish if you can; the person at the fish counter of your market or supermarket can tell you how to cook it if you are uncertain.

Try to have fish at least once a week—your insides will be grateful.

The possibilities for fish are endless:

Trout, herring, or mackerel, grilled or baked with a little butter or margarine on top

Cod, halibut, or haddock steaks baked in the oven, or cooked in foil on the broiler

Smoked fish (kippers or smoked haddock, for example) cooked in the oven with a little bit of water to keep them from becoming dry

## VEGETABLES

Be adventurous! You really don't need to exist on french fries, baked beans, frozen peas, and canned sweet corn. There are a whole lot of other vegetables out there—like these, for example:

| | |
|---|---|
| *Artichokes* | *Kale* |
| *Beans* | *Leeks* |
| *Beets* | *Mushrooms* |
| *Broccoli* | *Onions* |
| *Brussels sprouts* | *Parsnips* |
| *Cabbage* | *Peppers* |
| *Carrots* | *Spinach* |
| *Cauliflower* | *Spring greens* |
| *Celery* | *Zucchini* |

And this is just what you might expect to find during the year in an ordinary produce shop. A large supermarket or a farmer's market may have a more exotic selection.

You don't need to boil vegetables to death, either. You can steam them (in an inexpensive steamer basket that fits in a saucepan—available in most houseware shops), bake them in the oven, braise them gently in a little butter or margarine in a covered ovenproof dish, serve them chopped with butter and ground black pepper . . . almost any way you can think of.

If you have an unappetizing assortment of cold leftover vegetables lurking at the back of the fridge, try the following ideas.

### Stir-Fry Vegetables

Use any leftover vegetables, chopped fairly small, to which you might add some bean sprouts, cooked macaroni or spaghetti, and tofu cut into small cubes. Fry them all together in a small amount of oil until heated through, adding a few drops of tamari to enhance the flavor.

### Vegetable Pie

Fry all the leftover vegetables together for a minute or two, put them into an ovenproof dish, cover with a cheese sauce, and top with pastry (frozen puff pastry is ideal). Cook until the pastry is a light brown color, following the cooking instructions on the packet of pastry.

### SALADS

Salads are ideal to add to any main dish, or to eat on their own, or to take to work in a plastic container. Here are some suggestions for basic salads, which you can have with salad dressings or on their own:

*Kidney bean, onion, and chopped ham*
*Diced beet root, grated carrot, and watercress*
*Cottage cheese, nuts, and canned peaches*
*Watercress, celery, apple, and apricot*

*Homemade coleslaw with anything you like*

*Pasta, tuna, and cheese*

*Diced cooked potato, tuna, and peas*

*Cauliflower, sliced leeks, and kidney beans*

*Mixed beans*

*Grated carrot and grapes*

*Sliced zucchini, French-cut green beans, and apple*

*Sprout salad (alfalfa, clover, etc.) (make certain that they come from an uncontaminated source)*

*Sliced tomato and onion with black pepper*

*White cabbage with raisins and peanuts*

*Rice-based salads, adding anything you like*

*Cooked green lentils, with raw onions, mushrooms, and grated carrot*

Stop when your imagination runs out!

## SALAD DRESSINGS

As with salads themselves, you can be infinitely creative with the dressings. Here are just a few ideas:

*Yogurt with a teaspoon of dried mint and a tablespoon of lemon juice*

*2 tablespoons vinegar, 4 tablespoons sunflower oil, 1 teaspoon dried mustard (or 1 teaspoon prepared mustard), 2 teaspoons sugar, salt and pepper*

*2 tablespoons lemon juice, 3 tablespoons sunflower oil, 1 tablespoon honey, seasoning*

*Yogurt with wine vinegar and garlic*

*Mashed tofu with garlic and lemon juice (add more lemon juice or water if too thick)*

*Mashed tofu with oil, lemon juice, honey, and dry mustard (add more lemon juice or water if too thick)*

# Hummus

*8 oz. chick peas soaked overnight and cooked (much more quickly in a pressure cooker) or a 14 oz. can, drained (keep the liquid from cooked or drained chick peas)*

*1 clove garlic, crushed*

*1 tablespoon tahini (sesame butter)*

*3 tablespoons sunflower oil*

*2 tablespoons lemon juice*

Put drained chick peas in blender or food processor with all the other ingredients and blend until smooth. If necessary, add some of the drained liquid until the hummus has the consistency of soft whipped cream. (Make it stiffer for filling sandwiches.)

## BREAD, DOUGH, AND PASTRY

If you can eat wheat, you should have no problem finding whole wheat bread and flour. If you can't eat wheat, here are some recipes for nonwheat bread, dough and pastry.

The first few recipes are made using one of the gluten-free flours, and the last ones use rice flour, millet flour, and buckwheat. If you experiment with different sorts of wheat-free flour, you should soon find one that suits you best.

If you have a convection oven and are using gluten-free flour, follow these guidelines provided by the manufacturer:

As convection ovens can vary from one model to another only guidelines can be given. Generally speaking, temperatures of 20 degrees below those of an ordinary oven and baking times of up to one-third less should be effective. Baked food should be light golden brown when ready to take out of the oven. Overbaking will make the food too dry. A certain amount of trial and error will probably be needed to obtain best results in individual convection ovens. All gluten-free flours are suitable for baking in convection ovens if lower temperatures and shorter baking times are used.

## Gluten-free Wheat Bread WF

This bread, and the brown bread that follows, take only a couple of minutes to prepare for the oven and do not need to be left to rise. However, amounts must be carefully weighed out and not guessed.

*10 oz. gluten-free flour*
*1 packet instant yeast, supplied with flour, or similar*
*1 tablespoon sunflower oil*

*Exactly 8 fl. oz. warm water*

Put the flour in the bowl. Add the oil and sprinkle in the yeast. Stir. Pour in the water and mix to a creamy batter with a wooden spoon (do not use an electric beater). Turn into a greased one-pound loaf baking pan and immediately put into a 350° preheated oven to bake on the top shelf. When well-risen and crusty, after 1 hour, turn out of the pan and cool on a wire rack. Handle the loaf gently when it has baked as it must be left to "set." Cut when cold.

This recipe can also be used to make dough for a pizza crust. Instead of putting the newly mixed dough into a loaf pan, roll it out on a floured countertop until it looks like thick pastry. Transfer to a baking sheet. Cover with whatever ingredients you like—sliced tomatoes, mushrooms, ham, anchovies, and so on—and sprinkle with cheese and herbs, then leave to rise in a warm place for just 10 minutes. Put into the oven at 425°F on the top shelf for 12 to 15 minutes. Take out and serve hot.

## Shortbread Pastry WF

*8 oz. gluten-free pastry flour*
*2 pinches salt*
*3 oz. soft margarine*
*5 tablespoons cold water*

Mix the flour with the salt in a mixing bowl. Rub in the margarine until the mixture resembles bread crumbs. Add the water and mix to a sticky paste (the water releases the binder from the flour). Knead gradually, adding only a very small amount of extra flour, until one ball of dough has formed and the bowl is clean.

This pastry is easiest to use for small items that can be cut out of rolled-out dough and lifted off the countertop with a spatula. For larger items such as pies and pastries the dough should be rolled out between sheets of wax paper or greaseproof paper. The top paper is then peeled off and the pastry turned upside down over the dish, allowing the backing sheet to peel off. Any excess should be trimmed off with a knife and any breaks can be pressed together. The top pastry crust should then be rolled out in the same way and dropped on to the filled pie.

If preferred, the bottom part of pies can be pressed out with the fingers until the dish is neatly lined.

Bake for about 20 minutes at 425°F.

## Banana Bread WF

*6 oz. gluten-free flour*

*1 teaspoon wheat-free baking powder*

*2 oz. rice flour*

*a pinch of salt*

*2 oz. soft margarine*

*2 oz. soft brown sugar*

*1 egg, beaten*

*rind of 1 lemon, finely grated*

*1 medium-sized banana, mashed*

Put the flour, rice flour baking powder, and salt into a bowl. Mix well. Rub in the margarine with the fingers. Stir in the sugar, egg, lemon rind, and mashed banana. Spoon into a greased and floured small loaf pan. Bake for 45 to 50 minutes until light brown. Turn out of the pan and leave to cool on a wire rack. When cold serve thickly sliced and spread with butter or margarine. Store in plastic and eat within two days.

## Simple Banana Loaf WF

*7 oz. millet flour*

*2 teaspoons wheat-free baking powder (see page 233)*

*½ teaspoon baking soda*

*2½ oz. margarine*

*4½ oz. superfine sugar*

*4 ripe bananas, mashed*

*2 eggs*

Sift the millet flour, baking powder, and baking soda together. Rub in the margarine until well-mixed. Add the sugar and bananas. Mix well. Beat the eggs and add them to the other ingredients. Mix again. Grease a two-pound loaf pan with margarine. Turn mixture into the pan and bake for 1 hour at 375°F. Turn out on a wire rack to cool.

## Buckwheat Loaf WF

*1 tablespoon dried yeast*
*1 teaspoon brown sugar*
*½ cup warm water*
*3 oz. potato flour*
*2 oz. cornmeal*
*1 oz. soy flour*
*1 oz. buckwheat flour*
*½ teaspoon salt*

Mix the dried yeast, sugar, and warm water and leave in a warm place for 15 minutes. Sift the flours into a bowl and add the salt. Stir the yeast and liquid mixture and pour onto the flour mixture. Beat well with a wooden spoon to get rid of the lumps and to give a creamy consistency. Pour into a one-pound loaf pan and leave to stand for 5 minutes. Bake at 350°F for about 1 hour until well-risen and crusty. Remove from the pan and bake upside down for an extra 10 minutes. Turn out onto a wire rack to cool.

## Crackers WF
### (Makes about eight large, crisp crackers.)

*½ oz. rice bran*
*a pinch of salt*
*3½ oz. gluten-free flour*
*1 oz. soft margarine*
*3 tablespoons cold water*

Put the rice bran into a bowl with the salt and flour. Mix well. Add the margarine and rub in with the fingers until mixture resembles fine bread crumbs. Add the cold water and mix into one large lump of dough. Roll out (using more flour as needed) onto a thin sheet of dough. Cut into about eight rectangles (or sixteen smaller rectangles if preferred). Lift onto ungreased baking sheet with a spatula and prick squares all over with a fork. Bake for approximately 15 minutes at 450°F. Take crackers off the baking sheets with a spatula. Leave to cool and crisp on a wire rack.

When cold, store in an airtight container. Use them instead of bread—spread them with butter or margarine or top them with ingredients of your choice to make an open-faced sandwich.

## Chapati (Indian Bread) WF
### (Makes four)

*2 heaped tablespoons gluten-free flour*
*a pinch of salt*
*3 teaspoons sunflower oil*
*exactly 2 tablespoons cold water*
*sunflower oil for frying*

Put all of the ingredients into a bowl and mix to a paste. Use more of the flour to knead. Divide the dough into four balls and roll out thinly, using more flour. Heat, but do not grease, a griddle or heavy-based frying pan. Cook the chapati on both sides for about one minute or until crisp. When ready to use, heat a little oil in a frying pan. Fry quickly on both sides for a few seconds, just to recrisp them. Stack on a plate after draining on kitchen paper. Serve with curry and rice.

If you can eat wheat, chapatis can be made using special chapati flour, in which case you should follow the directions on the packet. You can also use this recipe:

*7 oz. whole grain flour*
*5 fl. oz. warm water*
*½ teaspoon salt*

Mix the flour and salt together, add the warm water, and mix to a dough. Knead well, then cover and leave for 30 minutes. Break off a piece of dough the size of a large walnut and, using plenty of flour, roll into a circle about 8 inches in diameter. Thoroughly heat a large, slightly oiled frying pan and cook the chapati until it is brown. Turn it over and cook on the other side. Repeat with the rest of the dough. Keep the chapatis warm until ready to serve.

## Date and Walnut Loaf WF

*8 oz. chopped dates*
*1 teaspoon baking soda*
*a pinch of salt*
*1 cup hot water*
*10 oz. rice flour*
*1 teaspoon wheat-free baking powder (see below)*
*4 oz. margarine*
*2 oz. shelled walnuts, chopped*
*4 oz. soft brown sugar*
*1 egg*

Place dates, baking soda, and salt in a bowl and pour the hot water over the top. Leave to cool. Sift the flour with the baking powder twice. Rub the margarine into the flour. Drain the dates and mix them into the flour along with the walnuts and sugar. Beat the egg and add to the flour mixture. Grease a two-pound loaf pan, fill with the mixture and bake for 1½ hours at 350°F. Turn out on to a wire tray to cool. Currants or raisins can be substituted for dates. This loaf cuts much better if left for a day.

## Tortillas WF
### (Makes about 6)

*4 oz. cornmeal*
*cold water to mix*

Put the cornmeal into a bowl and gradually add water to make a firm dough while you mix. Break off pieces of the dough and roll them out as thin as you can, between sheets of wax paper.

Heat a griddle or heavy-based frying pan and cook the tortillas for one minute on each side, without greasing. Use instead of bread with meals.

## Tacos WF

Make as for tortillas and, while still warm from cooking, fold lightly in half. Leave to cool on a wire rack. Stuff with salad vegetables or any sandwich fillings.

## Homemade Wheat-Free Baking Powder WF

*2 oz. rice flour*
*2 oz. baking soda*
*4½ oz. cream of tartar*

Sift the ingredients together at least three times. Store in an airtight container in a dry place. If you use this baking powder instead of standard baking powder, increase the amount by 50 percent; that is, if recipe calls for 2 teaspoons standard baking powder, use 3 teaspoons homemade powder.

### CAKES AND COOKIES

This section has recipes for cakes and cookies that do not contain wheat.

## Basic Plain Cake WF
### (You can add various flavorings.)

*2 oz. margarine*
*2 oz. sugar*
*1 egg*
*4 oz. gluten-free flour*
*1 teaspoon wheat-free baking powder*
*flavoring of your choice*

Grease and flour a one-pound loaf pan. Put all ingredients in a bowl, including the flavoring you have chosen, and mix to a soft, creamy consistency. If you think batter is too stiff, add a little cold milk. Put the mixture into the prepared loaf pan and bake for the first 25 to 30 minutes at 375°F, then for another 20 to 25 minutes at 350°F to cook the center. Let the cake cool in the pan for a minute and then place on a wire rack to cool. If you wish, you can sprinkle the top of the cake with granulated sugar before you put it in the oven.

Do not overbake this type of cake or it will be too dry. The actual baking time depends on the type of flavoring used:

*Carob:* add 2 heaped teaspoons carob powder. Use the shortest cooking time

*Chocolate:* add 2 heaping teaspoons cocoa

*Coffee:* add 2 slightly heaped teaspoons instant coffee

*Ginger:* add 1 heaped teaspoon dried ginger

*Lemon:* add the finely grated rind of one small lemon

*Orange:* add the finely grated rind of one orange

*Spice:* add 1 heaped teaspoon mixed spice

*Vanilla:* add a few drops of vanilla essence or flavoring

## Basic Fruit Cake Mix WF

*2 oz. sugar*
*2 oz. soft margarine*
*2 eggs*
*4 oz. gluten-free flour*
*½ teaspoon wheat-free baking powder*
*rind of ½ lemon, finely grated*
*4 oz. dried fruit (currants, raisins, cherries, apricots, according to taste)*

Grease and flour a one-pound loaf pan. Put all the ingredients into a mixing bowl, except the dried fruit. Mix until it is a soft dropping consistency. If it is too heavy, add a little milk and beat again. Stir in the fruit. Sprinkle the top with a little sugar if you wish. Bake for 30 minutes at 375°F and then either move the cake down one shelf or lower the heat to 350°F. Bake for another 30 minutes. Leave to cool in the pan for a minute or two and then turn out on to a wire rack to finish cooling. When cold, store in an airtight container. Eat within a week of baking.

## Fruit Cookies WF

*1 oz. polyunsaturated margarine*
*2 oz. ground rice*
*½ eating apple, finely grated*
*1 tablespoon brown sugar*
*1 slightly heaped tablespoon dried fruit*
*3 pinches mixed spice*
*grated rind of ¼ orange or lemon*

Put margarine and ground rice into a bowl and blend with a fork. Add the apple, sugar, fruit, spice, and rind. Mix with a wooden spoon until the dough forms one ball. Grease a baking sheet with margarine and drop spoons of the mixture on to it. Flatten slightly with the back of a teaspoon or a knife. Bake above the center of the oven for about 20 to 25 minutes at 450°F. Allow to cool on the baking sheet for 2 or 3 minutes and then remove to a wire cooling rack, using a spatula. As they grow cold, the cookies will crisp. Eat within a day of baking.

## Fruit and Nut Cookies WF

Make as for fruit cookies, but add 1 tablespoon of chopped walnuts, almonds, or hazelnuts.

## Ginger Snaps WF

*4 oz. gluten-free flour*
*½ teaspoon wheat-free baking powder*
*1 level teaspoon dried ginger*

*3 pinches powdered cloves (optional)*
*1 oz. soft margarine*
*2 oz. sugar*
*½ of a beaten egg*
*2 tablespoons golden syrup*

Put the flour, ginger, and ground cloves into a basin and mix well. Beat the margarine to a light cream. Add the sugar and beat again. Next, beat in the egg and syrup. Add the dry ingredients and mix to a very stiff paste. Knead, using more flour, and divide into about 16 balls. Roll each ball between your palms, put onto greased baking sheets, and flatten out to about 1¾ inches. Bake for about 12 to 15 minutes at 350°F. When a light golden color, put onto a wire rack to cool. Sprinkle with a little caster sugar and store in an airtight container.

## Plain Cookies WF
### (Makes about 20 large cookies)

*8 oz. gluten-free flour*
*1 teaspoon wheat-free baking powder*
*2 oz. soft margarine*
*2 oz. sugar*
*1 egg*

Cream the margarine and sugar. Beat in the egg. Add the flour and mix until it forms one ball of dough. Knead, using more of the flour and a little cold water if too stiff. Roll out the dough to about 1 inch thickness and cut into shapes with cutters or divide up with a sharp knife. Use a spatula to place on ungreased baking sheets. Prick with a fork and bake until pale gold—about 15 minutes at 400°F. Cool on a wire rack. Sprinkle with caster sugar and store in an airtight container.

This is a very useful basic cookie recipe—the cookies can be flavored, iced, sandwiched, topped, and so on. You can add the following flavorings:

*Chocolate:* add 1 heaped teaspoon of cocoa to the flour

*Cinnamon:* add ½ teaspoon cinnamon to the flour

*Coffee:* add 1 heaped teaspoon instant coffee to the flour

*Lemon:* add the finely grated rind of half a lemon

*Orange:* add the finely grated rind of one orange

*Spice:* add ½ teaspoon mixed spices to the flour

### Rich Chocolate Cake WF

*7 oz. gluten-free flour*
*1 teaspoon wheat-free baking powder*
*2 level tablespoons cocoa*
*5 oz. fine sugar*
*2 tablespoons molasses*
*2 eggs*
*5 tablespoons vegetable oil*
*5 tablespoons milk*

Sift the flour and cocoa into a mixing bowl. Add the sugar and mix well. In a smaller bowl, put the molasses, eggs, oil, and milk. Stir for a minute until blended well. Grease two 7-inch round sponge pans and flour them. Add the contents of the small bowl to the large one and mix well to form a shiny brown batter. Pour into the two prepared pans. Bake for 45 to 50 minutes at 300°F. When they are ready, the cakes will have shrunk slightly away from the side of the pans and when pressed lightly, they will spring back. Leave the cake to cool in the pan for a few minutes, then place on a wire rack to cool. Sandwich together with butter icing or jam. Store in an airtight container.

## DESSERTS

Fruit is a good way of getting dietary fiber, so try to eat plenty. Even if citrus fruits (oranges, lemons, grapefruit, and limes) disagree with you, there is still a great range available:

| | |
|---|---|
| Apples | Melons |
| Apricots | Nectarines |
| Blackberries | Passion fruit |
| Black currants | Peaches |
| Grapes | Pears |
| Guavas | Pineapple |
| Kiwi fruit | Plums |
| Lychees | Raspberries |
| Mangoes | Rhubarb |

The recipes that follow are all easy to shop for and quick to prepare. Most of them are high in fiber.

## Baked Apples

*1 baking apple per person*
*filling of your choice*
*sugar or honey to sweeten*

Remove the core from the apple, enlarge the hole slightly more, and fill with anything you like, such as

*Nuts*

*Dried chopped apricots*

*Raisins*

*Canned pineapple cubes*

*Mashed banana*

*Crushed pineapple*

*Blackberries*

*Raspberries*

Put on a flat ovenproof dish, add a small quantity of water, sprinkle with sugar or cover with about a tablespoon of thin honey, and bake in a moderate oven until the apple is just soft—about 30 minutes.

## Baked Pears

*1 to 2 pears per person*
*light honey*
*lemon juice*
*½ teaspoon ground cinnamon or ginger*

Cut the pears into halves or quarters and remove the core. Place in a flat ovenproof dish and cover with honey, a little lemon juice, and a sprinkling of ground cinnamon or ginger.

## Banana Dessert
**(You can use almost any other fruits for this dessert.)**

*1 lb. tofu*
*1 or 2 ripe bananas (or other fruit)*
*2 tablespoons honey*
*a few drops of vanilla essence or flavoring*

Blend the ingredients together, pour into a bowl, and serve well chilled.

## Carob Whip

*½ oz. corn flour*
*½ oz. carob powder*
*3 tablespoons sugar*
*1 egg, beaten*
*1 cup milk*
*yogurt or whipped double cream*
*1 oz. chopped mixed nuts*

Mix the corn flour, carob powder, sugar, and eggs together with enough of the milk to make a smooth paste. Heat the rest of the milk in a saucepan. When it is almost boiling, pour over the carob mixture, stirring all the time. Return to the saucepan and bring to a boil, stirring all the time. Boil for about a minute, then

leave to cool. Fold the yogurt or whipped cream into the cooled
mixture, add half the nuts, pour into a serving bowl, sprinkle the
rest of the nuts on top, and leave to chill.

## Crumble Topping for Fruit
### (For those who can eat wheat)

*6 oz. flour (or 4 oz. flour and 2 oz. oatmeal or All Bran)*
*3 oz. butter or margarine*
*2 to 3 oz. sugar*

Mix all ingredients in a mixer or food processor until it looks
like large bread crumbs. Sprinkle generously over fruit that is
already stewed and sweetened, and cook in a moderate oven for 10
to 15 minutes until the crumble is a pale brown color. It is a good
idea to make a hole in the topping so that the steam can escape,
which prevents the fruit from spilling over.

## Crumble Topping for Fruit WF
### (For those who can't eat wheat)

*6 oz. ground rice*
*3 oz. butter or margarine*
*2 oz. sugar*

—OR—
*6 oz. ground rice*
*2 oz. cooking almonds or oatmeal*
*2 oz. brown sugar*

Mix all the ingredients together until they resemble large
bread crumbs and sprinkle a good layer over stewed fruit. Cook as
in the previous recipe.

## Dried Fruit Compote

Buy a packet of dried fruit (usually a mixture of dried apples, prunes,
apricots, and peaches). Leave to soak in water for a few hours until

tender. (It will take less time if you bring the water to a boil first.) Can be eaten cold or heated, with sugar or yogurt, or just as it is.

## Fruit Brulée

*soft fruit (raspberries, sliced bananas, stewed apples, canned peaches, or any fruit you like)*
*whipping cream*
*brown sugar*

Place the fruit in an ovenproof dish, cover with whipped cream and a good sprinkling of brown sugar. Place under a hot grill until the sugar bubbles and melts (don't let it burn). Serve immediately.

## Fruit Jello

Make a jello according to the instructions, add fresh chopped or canned fruit, and leave in the fridge to set. If you put some of it into a plastic bowl with a lid, you can easily take it to work. (But don't let it become warm, or it will melt all over everything!)

## Instant Fruit Pie

Buy a ready-made pie crust from your grocer or supermarket (sweet-flavored rather than plain, if possible). Fill with stewed fruit and decorate with cream or yogurt.

## Crêpes

Use the recipes on pages 222–23 and serve with lemon juice and sugar or filled with stewed fruit.

## Raspberry Whip

*1 lb. raspberries (or any other soft fruit)*
*10 oz. tofu*
*sugar to taste*

Cook raspberries in a very little water with the sugar until just soft. Leave to cool. Liquefy in blender or food processor with the tofu until smooth. Serve chilled.

## Sliced Oranges

*1 to 2 oranges per person*
*sugar*
*small amount of water*

Peel the oranges, slice them, and lay them out in a flat dish. Dissolve about 2 oz. of sugar in about ½ cup water and heat until melted. It should taste just pleasantly sweet, not sickly. When cool, cover the sliced oranges with the sugar syrup and serve chilled.

## Rice Pudding

Since the days of Victorian literature, rice pudding has gotten bad press, but if you are willing to put childhood memories behind you and rethink previous judgment, you may have a pleasant surprise.

*4 oz. short-grain brown rice*
*1½ pints milk*
*2 oz. butter*
*3 oz. vanilla sugar (or vanilla pod)*
*2 eggs, well beaten*
*nutmeg to grate*

Cook the rice very gently in the milk for about 10 minutes. Add the butter and sugar, stirring carefully. Remove from the heat, allow to cool a little, then stir in the beaten eggs. Put the mixture into a well-greased baking dish, sprinkle with nutmeg (freshly grated nutmeg tastes much nicer than ground nutmeg), and bake for 30 to 40 minutes at 300°F. Serve plain or with jam, golden syrup, or honey.

## Yogurt with Fruit

Make your own yogurt or buy a large carton of plain yogurt. Add some fresh or canned fruit and sweeten with honey.

DRINKS

There has to be more to life than endless cups of coffee! Herb teas are a good substitute, and you can keep one or two teabags concealed about your person for those occasions when you might be expected to drink coffee. Herb teas come in many flavors—peppermint, nettle, strawberry, chamomile, apple, orange, and so on. There are "daytime teas" to keep you awake and "night-time" teas to help you sleep. If you find their taste a bit sharp, add a teaspoon or two of honey.

## Carob and Banana Drink
**(You can substitute any other soft fruit: stewed apricots, raspberries, prunes, stewed black currants, and so on.)**

*1 pint milk*
*2 teaspoons thin honey*
*2 tablespoons carob powder*
*1 banana (or other fruit), peeled and sliced*

Mix ingredients together in a blender or food processor. Serve chilled.

## Homemade Lemonade

*3½ cups water*
*2 oz. sugar*
*½ teaspoon citric acid*
*1 lemon, cut in pieces*

Mix all the ingredients together in a blender or food processor. Strain. Leave to cool.

## Tomato Juice

*carton tomato juice*
*carton yogurt (or about 4 to 5 oz.)*
*½ cup apple juice*
*a few mint leaves (if available)*

Mix all the ingredients together in a blender or food processor. Serve chilled.

## Ginger Beer

*½ oz. fresh yeast*
*2 teaspoons ground ginger*
*1½ cups water*
*2 teaspoons sugar*

Mix all together in a jug or bowl and leave for 24 hours. Feed daily with 1 teaspoon of ground ginger and 1 teaspoon sugar. After seven days, strain the liquid through muslin or cheesecloth and put the solid residue to one side. Mix the strained liquid with 5 pints of cold water and the juice of two lemons. Dissolve 1½ lb. of sugar in hot water and mix well into the strained liquid. Pour into screwtop bottles and leave for one week before drinking. Divide the solid residue in half, add ½ oz. fresh yeast, 1½ cups water, 2 teaspoons ground ginger, 2 teaspoons sugar, and repeat as above. You now have the basis of a lifetime's supply of homemade ginger beer.

# *Appendix*

## Substitute Foods

### Grains

*Breakfast cereals:* Rice Krispies, puffed rice, oatmeal, some makes of muesli

*Corn:* wheat, rye, oats, barley

*Wheat-based breads and biscuits:* gluten-free bread, rye bread, rye crispbreads, oatcakes, rice cakes, rice crackers

*Wheat-based pasta:* pasta made with gluten-free flour; rice, rice noodles, buckwheat noodles, potatoes

*Wheat flour:* rice flour, potato flour, soy flour, rye flour, corn flour, buckwheat, millet, oats, oatmeal, arrowroot, tapioca, sago; sauces can be thickened with tapioca flour, potato flour, ground rice

### Dairy Products

Goat's milk may be suitable; yogurt may be suitable in small quantities; Lactaid or other lactose-free products, soy milk (calcium-fortified if possible), rice milk, Spectrum spread, Shedd's Willow Run

Spread, kosher spreads, sunflower spreads, clarified butter (ghee) are all possible alternatives.

## Vegetables and Fruits

*Citrus fruits:* almost any other fruit

*Corn oil or vegetable oil:* sunflower oil, safflower oil, soybean oil

*Potatoes:* rice, pasta, chapatis, yams, sweet potatoes

## Beverages

*Black tea or coffee:* herb teas, fruit juices, chicory drinks, vegetable drinks

*Tap water:* bottled spring water is an obvious substitute, but if you think tap water disagrees with you, you should see your doctor before eliminating it

*Yeast (in alcohol):* nonalcoholic drinks

## Snacks and Baking

*Baking powder:* mix together 35 g bicarbonate of soda, 70 g cream of tartar, and 70 g of arrowroot. Store in an airtight container and use 1½ teaspoons of this baking powder for 1 teaspoon of ordinary baking powder

*Chocolate:* carob, cocoa

*Flavorings:* cinnamon, nutmeg, parsley, paprika, celery salt, pepper, vanilla, carob

*Spreads:* spreadable fruit, honey

*Quick snacks:* sunflower seeds, sesame seed bars

*Yeast (in bread):* soda bread, tortillas, chapatis, unleavened breads

# *Other Resources*

## Helpful Websites & Addresses

**IBS Self Help Group: www.ibsgroup.org**
www.panix.com/~ibs

**International Foundation for Functional Gastrointestinal Disorders (IFFGD)**
P.O. Box 170864
Milwaukee, WI 53217
888-964-2001
www.iffgd.org

**IBS Support Group for Southern California**
2446 26th Street
Santa Monica, CA 90405
310-392-3010
www.geocities.com/Hollywood/Boulevard/2957/ibs.html

**IBS Bulletin and Review of International Research**
IBS Research Appeal
Central Middlesex Hospital Trust
Freepost TK 1409
Hampton Hill, Middlesex, TW12 1BR
England
www.ibsresearchupdate.org

# Index

# Other Ulysses Press Mind/Body/Spirit Books

**ANXIETY & DEPRESSION: A NATURAL APPROACH**
*2nd edition, Shirley Trickett, $10.95*
A step-by-step organic solution for preventing anxiety and conquering depression that puts the reader—not the drugs—in control.

**THE EASY GL DIET HANDBOOK: LOSE WEIGHT WITH THE REVOLUTIONARY GLYCEMIC LOAD PROGRAM**
*Dr. Fedon Alexander Lindberg, $10.00*
Using these more accurate and sensible GL scores, *The Easy GL Diet Handbook* offers a plan for healthy weight loss and reduced risk of diabetes that's easier to follow. It also includes numerous foods that the Atkins, South Beach, and GI diets wrongly consider "off-limits."

**FLIP THE SWITCH: 40 ANYTIME, ANYWHERE MEDITATIONS IN 5 MINUTES OR LESS**
*Eric Harrison, $10.95*
Specially designed meditations that fit any situation: idling at a red light, waiting for a computer to restart, or standing in line at the grocery store.

**HEPATITIS C**
*2nd edition, Beth Ann Petro Roybal, $13.95*
Addresses the rapidly changing status of hepatitis C with information on therapeutic strategies and the search for a cure.

**HOW MEDITATION HEALS: SCIENTIFIC EVIDENCE AND PRACTICAL APPLICATION**
*2nd edition, Eric Harrison, $14.95*
In straightforward, practical terms, *How Meditation Heals* reveals how and why meditation improves the natural functioning of the human body.

**IRRITABLE BLADDER & INCONTINENCE: A NATURAL APPROACH**
*Jennifer Hunt, $8.95*
This handy volume offers a simple yet powerful program for taking control of your life.

**THE LEPTIN BOOST DIET: UNLEASH YOUR FAT-CONTROLLING HORMONES FOR MAXIMUM WEIGHT LOSS**
*Scott Isaacs, M.D.*
A series of recent medical breakthroughs have confirmed what physicians suspected all along—obesity is a hormonal disorder. *The Leptin Boost Diet* transforms these findings into a unique and easy-to-follow weight-loss program.

**MIGRAINES: A NATURAL APPROACH**
*2nd edition, Sue Dyson, $12.95*
Offers easy-to-understand explanations and holistic treatments to this major health problem.

**PANIC ATTACKS: A NATURAL APPROACH**
*2nd edition, Shirley Trickett, $9.95*
Offers a completely natural mind/body treatment not provided by traditional therapies, including use of proper diet, relaxation and breathing exercises.

**KNOW YOUR BODY: THE ATLAS OF ANATOMY**
*2nd edition, Introduction by Emmet B. Keeffe, M.D., $14.95*
Provides a comprehensive, full-color guide to the human body.

**PORTABLE REIKI: EASY SELF-TREATMENTS FOR HOME, WORK AND ON THE GO**
*Tanmaya Honervogt, $14.95*
Presents do-it-yourself, step-by-step treatments for quick, effective Reiki healing—anytime, anyplace. The book's system is specially designed to help busy people release stress, improve health and restore personal energy.

**YOGA IN FOCUS: POSTURES, SEQUENCES AND MEDITATIONS**
*Jessie Chapman    Photographs by Dhyan, $14.95*
A yoga book unlike any other, *Yoga in Focus* could just as easily be a gift book as a tutorial. The presentation captures the very essence of yoga, combining perfectly positioned figures in meditative black-and-white photos.

*To order these books call 800-377-2542 or 510-601-8301, fax 510-601-8307, e-mail ulysses@ulyssespress.com, or write to Ulysses Press, P.O. Box 3440, Berkeley, CA 94703. All retail orders are shipped free of charge. California residents must include sales tax. Allow two to three weeks for delivery.*

# About the Authors

**Rosemary Nicol** lives in Somerset, England, and is married with four children. As well as the bestselling *Irritable Bowel Syndrome: A Natural Approach,* she is also the author of *Everything You Need to Know About Osteoporosis* and *Sleep Like a Dream—the Drug-Free Way.*

**William John Snape, Jr., M.D.**, is a leading gastroenterologist specializing in the treatment of functional gastrointestinal disorders. He has published numerous original articles on IBS in such medical journals as *Gastroenterology, American Journal of Digestive Disease,* and the *New England Journal of Medicine.* Dr. Snape, formerly associated with Harbor-UCLA Medical Center, is currently the Director of Gastrointestinal Motility at California Pacific Medical Center in San Francisco, California.